Clinical Electrocardiography
SELF-ASSESSMENT AND REVIEW

D1567709

Clinical Electrocardiography
SELF-ASSESSMENT AND REVIEW

Donald A. Underwood, M.D.
Head, Section of Electrocardiography
Department of Cardiology
The Cleveland Clinic Foundation
Cleveland, Ohio

W.B. SAUNDERS COMPANY
Harcourt Brace Jovanovich, Inc.
Philadelphia • London • Toronto • Montreal • Sydney • Tokyo

W.B. Saunders Company
Harcourt Brace & Company

The Curtis Center
Independence Square West
Philadelphia, Pennsylvania 19106

Library of Congress
Cataloging-in-Publication Data

Underwood, Donald A.
    Clinical electrocardiography: self-assessment and
review / Donald A. Underwood. — 1st ed.
        p.   cm.
    Includes index.
    ISBN 0-7216-6692-2
    1. Electrocardiography — Examinations and
questions.   I. Title.
    [DNLM: 1. Electrocardiography — examination
questions.   WG 18 U56c 1993]
RC683.5.E5U54   1993
616.1′207547 — dc20
DNLM/DLC   93-18060

Clinical Electrocardiography:
Self-Assessment and Review   ISBN 0-7216-6692-2

Printed in the United States of America.

Last digit is the print number: 9   8   7   6   5   4   3   2   1

Lee C. Underwood, M.D.
William L. Proudfit, M.D.
Royston C. Lewis, M.D.

Three great electrocardiographers
in the order I met them.

Contents

Introduction

The electrocardiogram is a clinical tool. Proper interpretation is dependent on multiple factors, among which is a high-quality tracing obtained on a high-fidelity machine that meets basic requirements for data acquisition. The electrocardiogram is best interpreted in light of broad clinical experience so that the effects of diseases encountered on it can be anticipated. The student needs to have adequate exposure to large numbers of tracings in multiple clinical settings as well as prompt feedback after an independent interpretation has been attempted. Interpretation and feedback either didactically or by way of the clinical arena are the basis of developing skill in the electrocardiographic laboratory.

This series of quizzes was developed in an attempt to reinforce the experience of the Cardiology Fellows at the Cleveland Clinic Foundation. The collection evolved over a period of years. The main goal was to offer an objective means for self-assessment about one's progress in electrocardiographic interpretation. As with all things in clinical medicine, the cornerstone of excellence is experience and exposure. This type of text cannot take the place of adequate time in the electrocardiographic laboratory or at the bedside. A complete reference text of electrocardiography is also essential. It can serve as a source of confidence, if most of the quizzes are completed with a high degree of agreement with the answer lists and as a means of identifying areas in which increased reading might be needed.

The format is fairly straightforward. A series of uninterpreted tracings are available for review. One or multiple diagnoses can be coded onto the answer sheet from the list of electrocardiographic possibilities, which can be found at the beginning of each exercise, and the answers compared with a brief description of each tracing, which emphasizes the important diagnostic points. Individual or group scoring can be done in a variety of ways but is not as important as the actual exercise of interpreting the electrocardiogram in an independent fashion and then getting instant feedback from the clinical description. (It probably will be easiest to use the text if copies of the code sheet and answer sheet are used instead of those bound in the book.)

You may not always agree; that is all right, as long as you can defend your conclusions through reading or experience. Good luck, and enjoy yourselves.

The same list of findings — the Electrocardiographic Diagnostic Coding Sheet — is used throughout this series of quizzes. Item entries should be in the same way that the electrocardiogram is interpreted. The sequence is not important and should reflect the pattern used by the individual doing the exercise. The electrocardiogram should be reviewed, appropriate points mentally noted, and the phrases or items that match these points entered onto the answer sheet.

All electrocardiograms are displayed in a standard three-channel fashion. There are four vertical panels of 2.5 seconds each, which correspond to lead groups I, II, and III: aV_R, aV_L, and aV_F; V_1 through V_3; and V_4 through V_6, respectively, from left to right.

In the following example, the patient is a 32-year-old woman with a history of rheumatic fever. The electrocardiogram shows notched P waves in lead II and a broadly negative terminal P wave component in lead V_1, which suggests left atrial enlargement. There is right axis deviation and an incomplete right bundle branch block plus $R' > S$ and T wave inversion in lead V_1. This is diagnostic of right ventricular hypertrophy. The inferior lead ST segment changes are nonspecific but represent definite abnormalities. This person should be coded for right ventricular hypertrophy (68), left atrial enlargement (63), incomplete right bundle branch block (54), and nonspecific ST-T wave changes (89). If a clinical diagnosis were going to be made, mitral stenosis or, more broadly, mitral valve disease (96) would be high on the list.

Use of the Electrocardiographic Diagnostic Coding Sheet and the Answer Sheet

1

Electrocardiographic Diagnostic Coding Sheet

General Features
1. Normal ECG
2. Normal ECG, variant
3. Misplaced leads
4. Electrical alternans

Sinus Rhythms
5. Normal sinus
6. Sinus tachycardia
7. Sinus bradycardia
8. Sinus arrhythmia
9. Sinus pause or arrest

Atrial Rhythms
10. Premature atrial contractions (PAC)
11. Aberrant PAC
12. Ectopic atrial rhythm
13. Atrial tachycardia with AV block
14. Atrial fibrillation
15. Atrial flutter
16. Multifocal atrial tachycardia
17. Dual atrial rhythms

AV Junctional Rhythms
18. Premature junctional beats (PJB)
19. Aberrant PJB
20. Junctional beat or rhythm
21. AV junctional rhythm with retrograde atrial activation
22. Supraventricular tachycardia

Ventricular Rhythms
23. Premature ventricular contractions (PVC), unifocal
24. PVC, multifocal
25. PVC, couplets or triplets
26. PVC, R-on-T phenomenon

27. Ventricular tachycardia
28. Idioventricular rhythm
29. Ventricular fibrillation
30. Ventricular escape beat or rhythm
31. Ventricular fusion beat or rhythm
32. Ventricular capture beat during VT
33. Torsade de pointes

Pacemaker Rhythms
34. Fixed rate
35. Demand
36. Atrial pacing
37. Ventricular pacing
38. Dual chamber pacing
39. Failure to sense
40. Failure to capture

AV Conduction Abnormalities
41. 1° AV block, or
42. Wenckebach (Mobitz I) AV block
43. 2° AV block (Mobitz II)
44. Fixed 2° AV block, 2:1, 4:1, etc.
45. Complete heart block
46. Variable AV block
47. Preexcitation (WPW)

AV-VA Interactions
48. Fusion beat
49. Echo beat
50. AV dissociation
51. Isorhythmic AV dissociation

Intraventricular Conduction Abnormalities
52. Left axis

53. Right axis
54. Incomplete RBBB
55. Complete RBBB
56. Incomplete LBBB
57. Complete LBBB
58. Anterior hemiblock
59. Posterior hemiblock
60. Nonspecific IVCD
61. Arrhythmia related aberrancy
62. Intermittent IVCD/BBB

Chamber Enlargement
63. Left atrial enlargement
64. Right atrial enlargement
65. Bi-atrial enlargement
66. LVH — voltage
67. LVH — voltage plus repolarization changes
68. RVH
69. Biventricular hypertrophy

Myocardial Infarction
Recent/Acute
70. Anteroseptal
71. Anterior
72. Lateral
73. Inferior
74. Posterior

Old/Uncertain Age
75. Anteroseptal
76. Anterior
77. Lateral
78. Inferior
79. Posterior

Repolarization Changes
80. Possible LV aneurysm
81. Non-W wave infarction

82. Early repolarization
83. Persistent juvenile T wave
84. ST-T wave changes of acute injury
85. ST-T wave changes of acute ischemia
86. ST-T wave changes of hypertrophy or altered intraventricular conduction (secondary repolarization changes)
87. ST-T wave changes of pericarditis
88. ST changes due to digitalis effect
89. Nonspecific ST-T wave changes
90. Postectopic T wave changes
91. Peaked T waves
92. Prolonged QT interval
93. Prominent U waves

Clinical Problems
94. Coronary artery disease
95. Congenital heart disease
96. Mitral valve disease
97. Hyperkalemia
98. Hypokalemia
99. Hypercalcemia
100. Hypocalcemia
101. Digitalis toxicity
102. CNS event
103. Motion artifact
104. Dextrocardia
105. Cardiac tamponade
106. Cardiac transplant
107. Chronic lung disease

ANSWER SHEET

Patient 1 — — — — — — — —

Patient 2 — — — — — — — —

Patient 3 — — — — — — — —

Patient 4 — — — — — — — —

Patient 5 — — — — — — — —

Patient 6 — — — — — — — —

Patient 7 — — — — — — — —

Patient 8 — — — — — — — —

Patient 9 — — — — — — — —

Patient 10 — — — — — — — —

Patient 11 — — — — — — — —

Patient 12 — — — — — — — —

Patient 13 — — — — — — — —

Patient 14 — — — — — — — —

Patient 15 — — — — — — — —

4

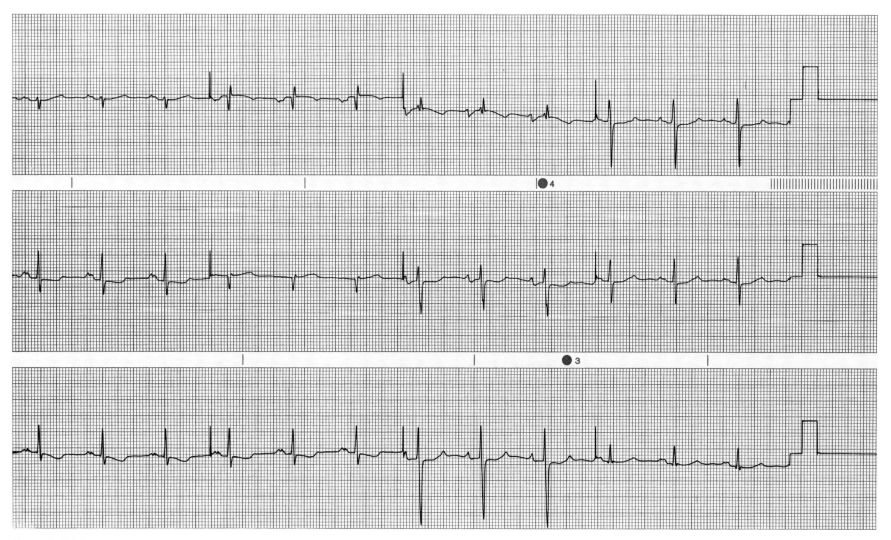

Example ECG

ANSWER SHEET
Example Patient

Example 1   68   63   54   89   96   ____   ____   ____

Exercise I

ANSWER SHEET
Exercise I

Patient 1 ⎯ ⎯ ⎯ ⎯ ⎯ ⎯ ⎯ ⎯

Patient 2 ⎯ ⎯ ⎯ ⎯ ⎯ ⎯ ⎯ ⎯

Patient 3 ⎯ ⎯ ⎯ ⎯ ⎯ ⎯ ⎯ ⎯

Patient 4 ⎯ ⎯ ⎯ ⎯ ⎯ ⎯ ⎯ ⎯

Patient 5 ⎯ ⎯ ⎯ ⎯ ⎯ ⎯ ⎯ ⎯

Patient 6 ⎯ ⎯ ⎯ ⎯ ⎯ ⎯ ⎯ ⎯

Patient 7 ⎯ ⎯ ⎯ ⎯ ⎯ ⎯ ⎯ ⎯

Patient 8 ⎯ ⎯ ⎯ ⎯ ⎯ ⎯ ⎯ ⎯

Patient 9 ⎯ ⎯ ⎯ ⎯ ⎯ ⎯ ⎯ ⎯

Patient 10 ⎯ ⎯ ⎯ ⎯ ⎯ ⎯ ⎯ ⎯

Patient 11 ⎯ ⎯ ⎯ ⎯ ⎯ ⎯ ⎯ ⎯

Patient 12 ⎯ ⎯ ⎯ ⎯ ⎯ ⎯ ⎯ ⎯

Patient 13 ⎯ ⎯ ⎯ ⎯ ⎯ ⎯ ⎯ ⎯

Patient 14 ⎯ ⎯ ⎯ ⎯ ⎯ ⎯ ⎯ ⎯

Patient 15 ⎯ ⎯ ⎯ ⎯ ⎯ ⎯ ⎯ ⎯

Electrocardiographic Diagnostic Coding Sheet

General Features
1. Normal ECG
2. Normal ECG, variant
3. Misplaced leads
4. Electrical alternans

Sinus Rhythms
5. Normal sinus
6. Sinus tachycardia
7. Sinus bradycardia
8. Sinus arrhythmia
9. Sinus pause or arrest

Atrial Rhythms
10. Premature atrial contractions (PAC)
11. Aberrant PAC
12. Ectopic atrial rhythm
13. Atrial tachycardia with AV block
14. Atrial fibrillation
15. Atrial flutter
16. Multifocal atrial tachycardia
17. Dual atrial rhythms

AV Junctional Rhythms
18. Premature junctional beats (PJB)
19. Aberrant PJB
20. Junctional beat or rhythm
21. AV junctional rhythm with retrograde atrial activation
22. Supraventricular tachycardia

Ventricular Rhythms
23. Premature ventricular contractions (PVC), unifocal
24. PVC, multifocal
25. PVC, couplets/triplets
26. PVC, R-on-T phenomenon

27. Ventricular tachycardia
28. Idioventricular rhythm
29. Ventricular fibrillation
30. Ventricular escape beat or rhythm
31. Ventricular fusion beat or rhythm
32. Ventricular capture beat during VT
33. Torsades de pointes

Pacemaker Rhythms
34. Fixed rate
35. Demand
36. Atrial pacing
37. Ventricular pacing
38. Dual chamber pacing
39. Failure to sense
40. Failure to capture

AV Conduction Abnormalities
41. 1° AV block
42. Wenckebach (Mobitz I) AV block
43. 2° AV block (Mobitz II)
44. Fixed 2° AV block, 2:1, 4:1, etc.
45. Complete heart block
46. Variable AV block
47. Preexcitation (WPW)

AV - VA Interactions
48. Fusion beat
49. Echo beat
50. AV dissociation
51. Isorhythmic AV dissociation

Intraventricular Conduction Abnormalities
52. Left axis

53. Right axis
54. Incomplete RBBB
55. Complete RBBB
56. Incomplete LBBB
57. Complete LBBB
58. Anterior hemiblock
59. Posterior hemiblock
60. Nonspecific IVCD
61. Arrhythmia related aberrancy
62. Intermittent IVCD/BBB

Chamber Enlargement
63. Left atrial enlargement
64. Right atrial enlargement
65. Bi-atrial enlargement
66. LVH - voltage
67. LVH - voltage plus repolarization changes
68. RVH
69. Biventricular hypertrophy

Myocardial Infarction

Recent/Acute
70. Anteroseptal
71. Anterior
72. Lateral
73. Inferior
74. Posterior

Old/Uncertain Age
75. Anteroseptal
76. Anterior
77. Lateral
78. Inferior
79. Posterior

Repolarization Changes
80. Possible LV aneurysm
81. Non-Q wave infarction

82. Early repolarization
83. Persistent juvenile T wave
84. ST-T wave changes of acute injury
85. ST-T wave changes of acute ischemia
86. ST-T wave changes of hypertrophy or altered intraventricular conduction (secondary repolarization changes)
87. ST-T wave changes of pericarditis
88. ST changes due to digitalis effect
89. Nonspecific ST-T wave changes
90. Postectopic T wave changes
91. Peaked T waves
92. Prolonged QT interval
93. Prominent U waves

Clinical Problems
94. Coronary artery disease
95. Congenital heart disease
96. Mitral valve disease
97. Hyperkalemia
98. Hypokalemia
99. Hypercalcemia
100. Hypocalcemia
101. Digitalis toxicity
102. CNS event
103. Motion artifact
104. Dextrocardia
105. Cardiac tamponade
106. Cardiac transplant
107. Chronic lung disease

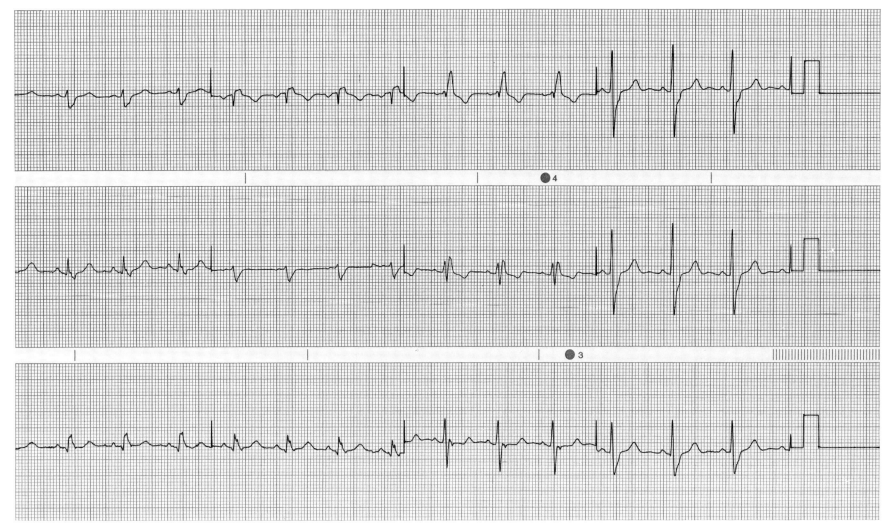

Exercise I, Patient 1

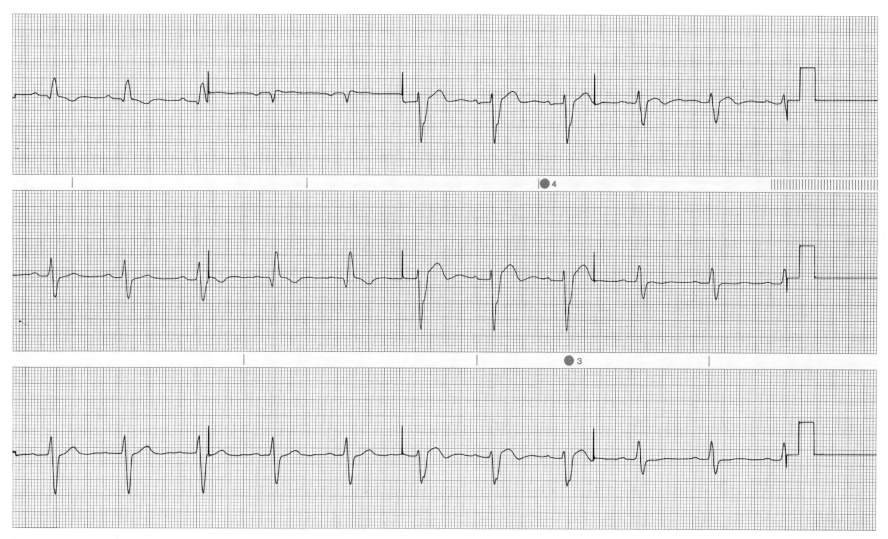

Exercise I, Patient 2

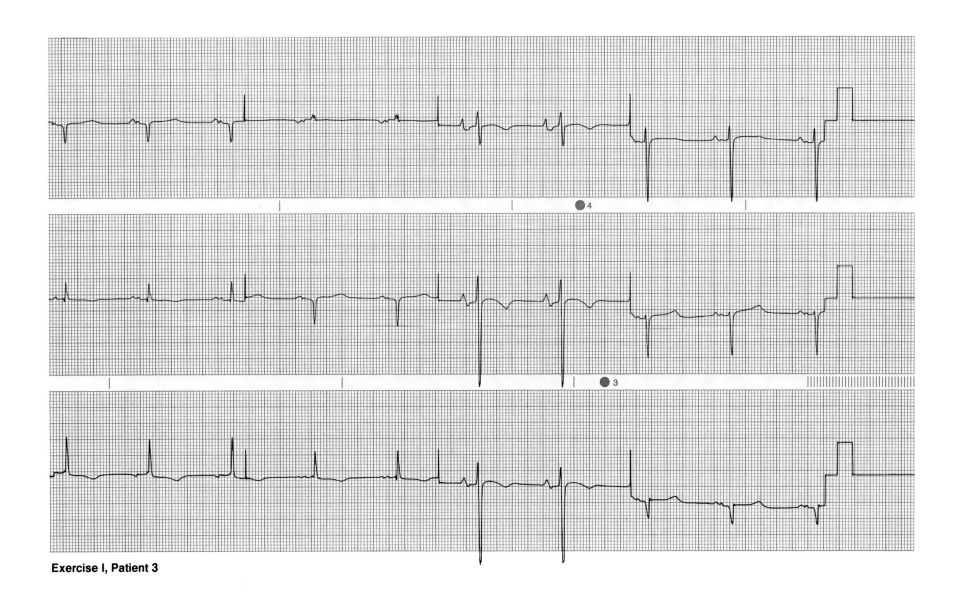

Exercise I, Patient 3

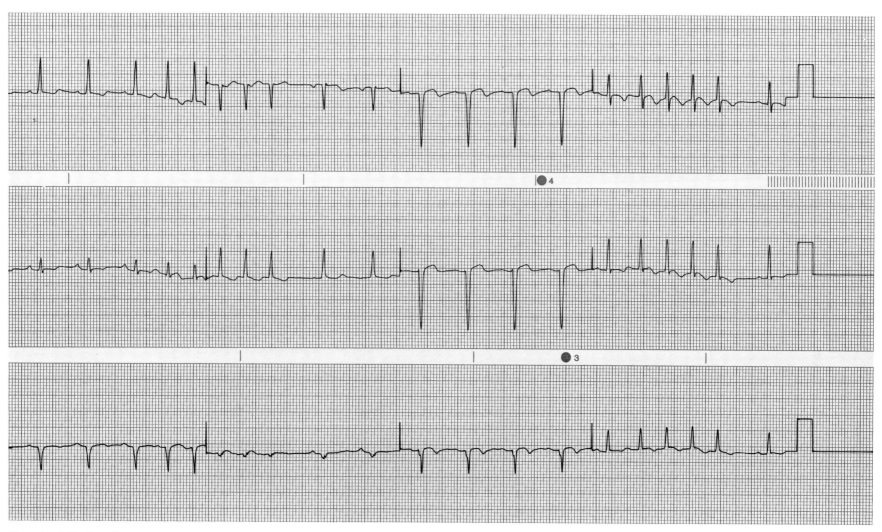

Exercise I, Patient 4

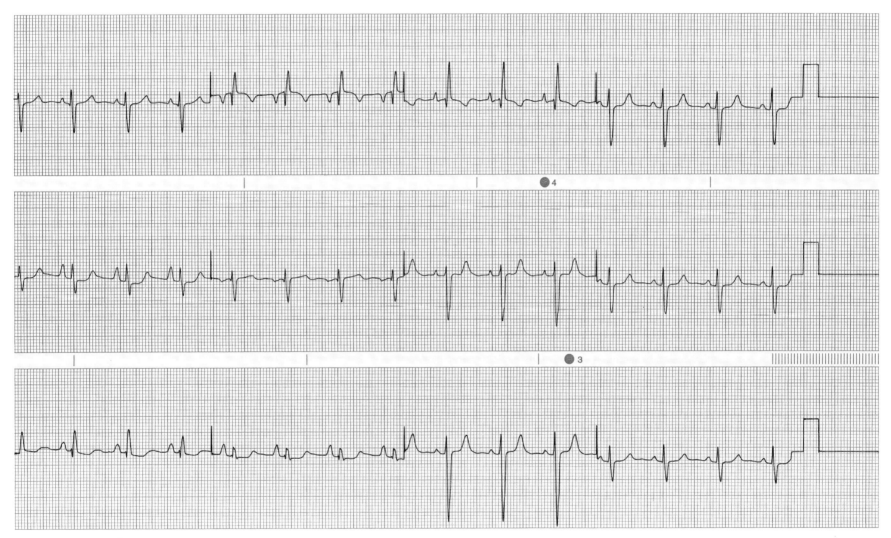

Exercise I, Patient 5

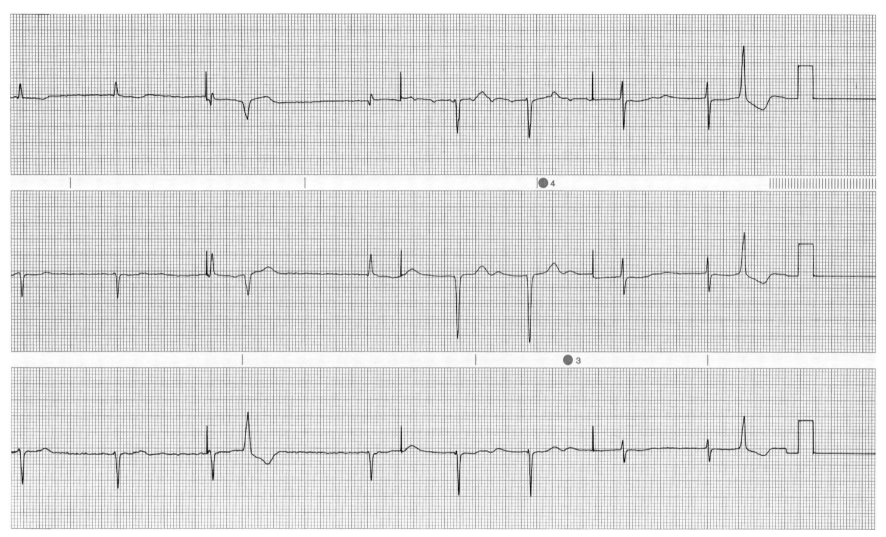

Exercise I, Patient 6

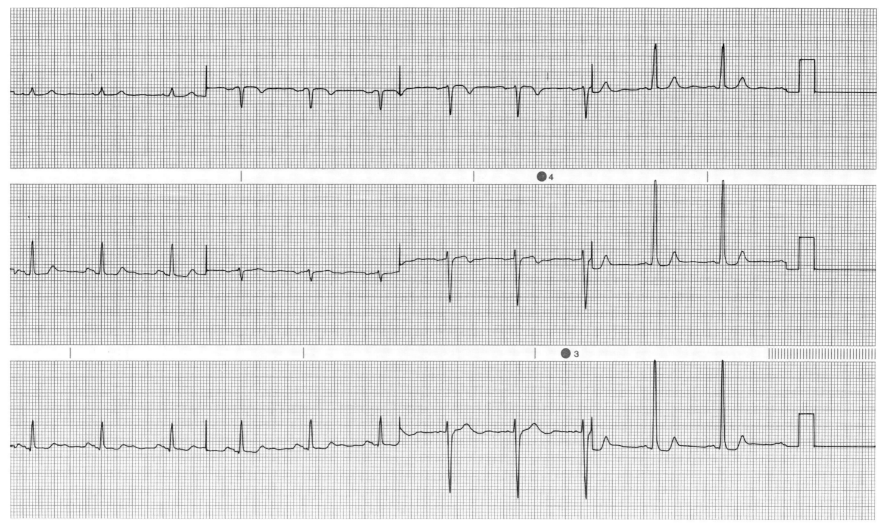

Exercise I, Patient 7

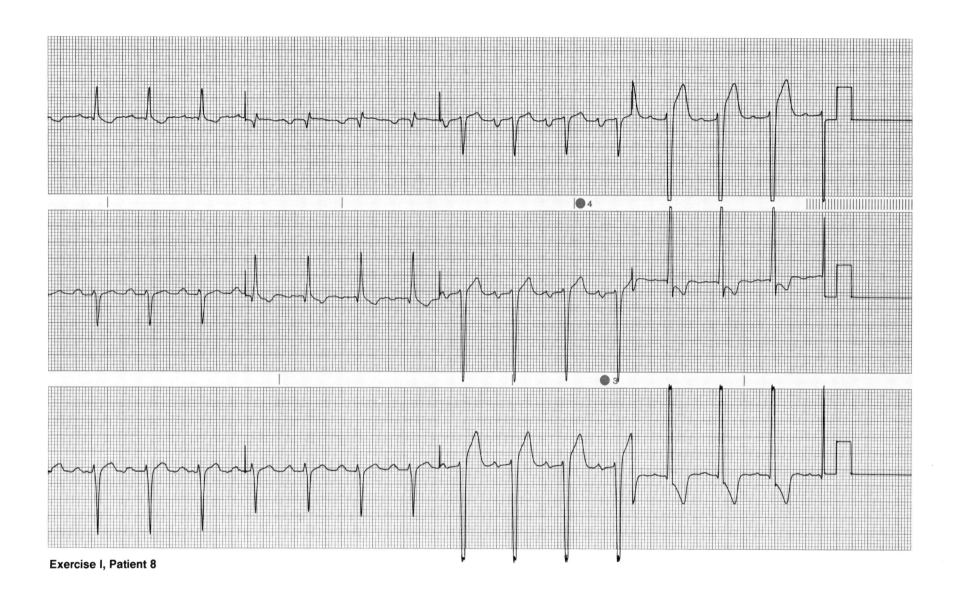

Exercise I, Patient 8

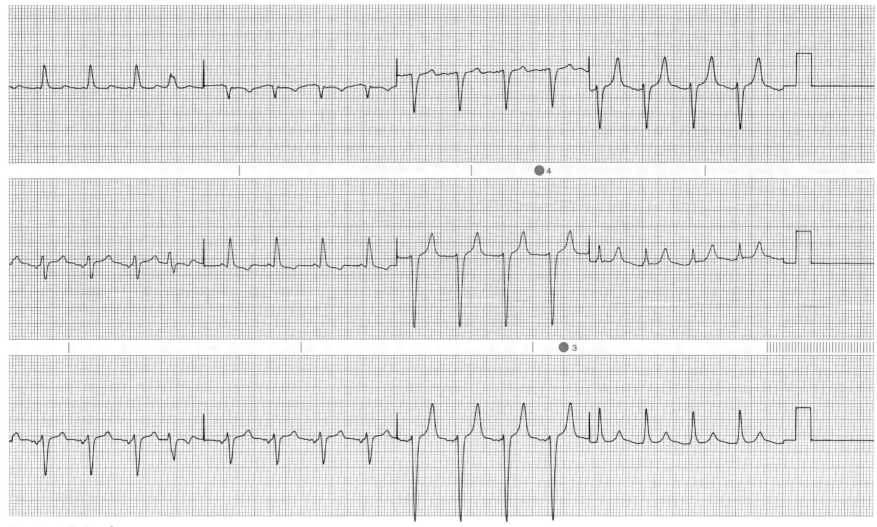

Exercise I, Patient 9

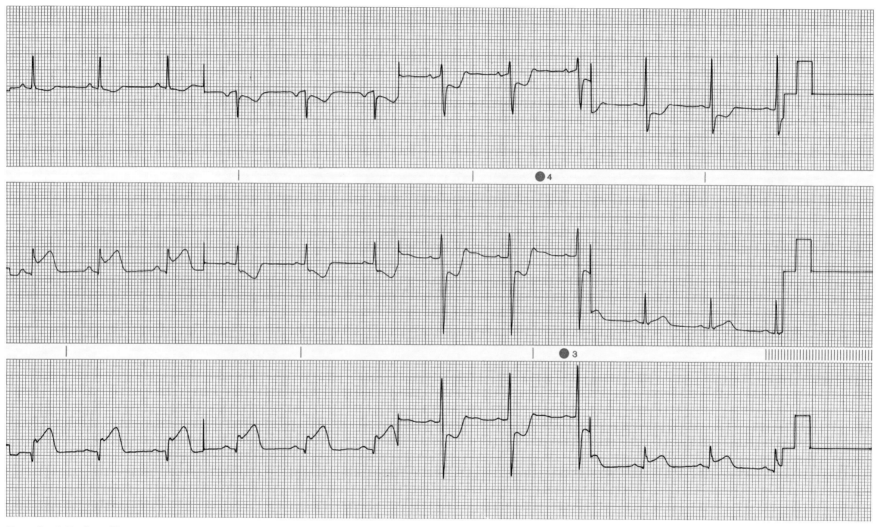

Exercise I, Patient 10

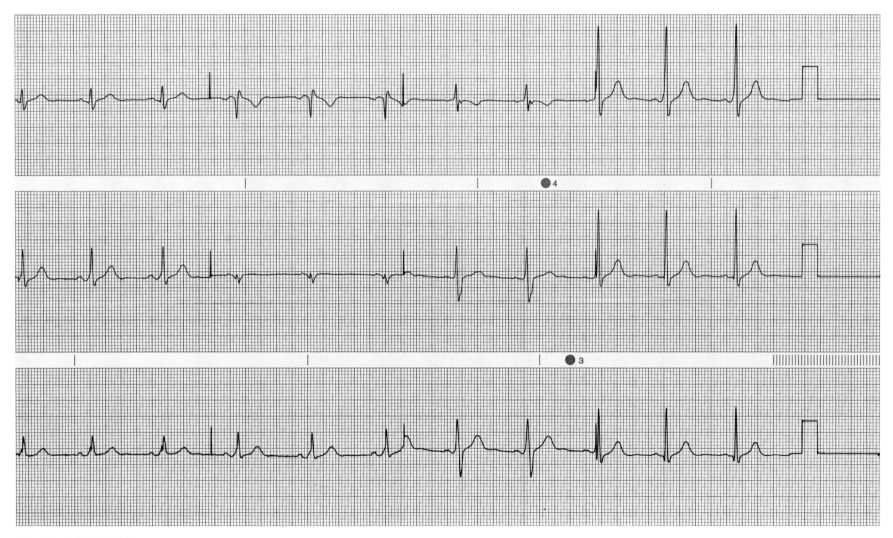

Exercise I, Patient 11

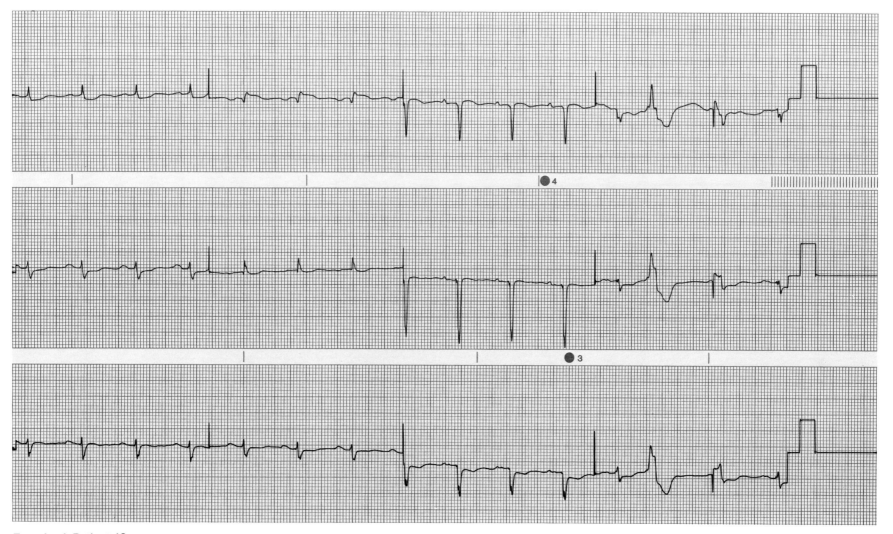

Exercise I, Patient 12

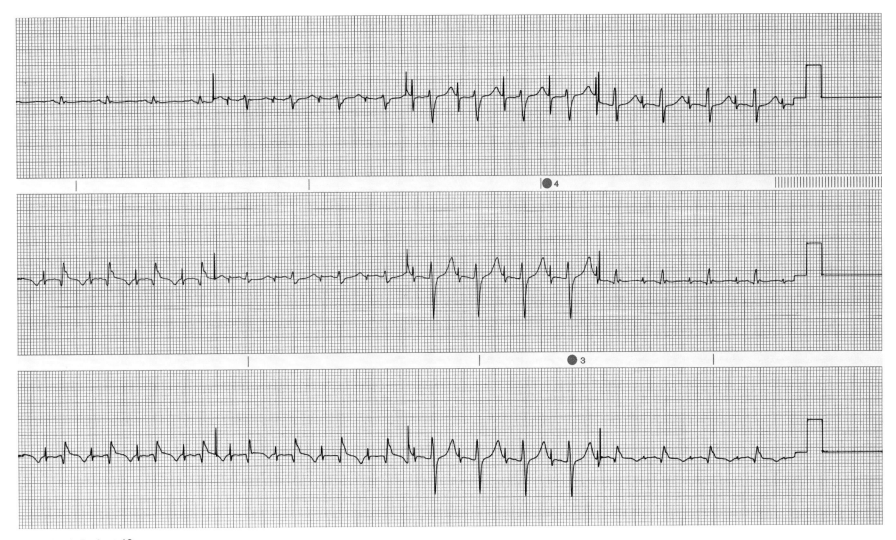

Exercise I, Patient 13

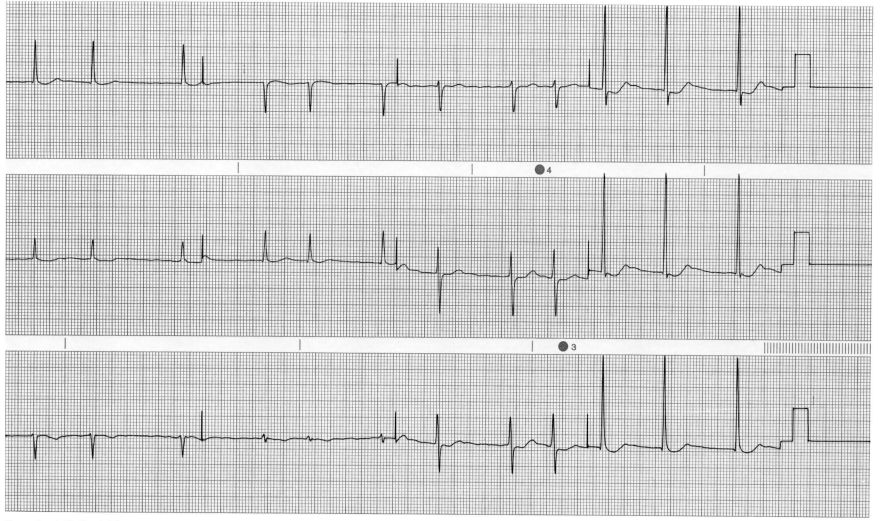

Exercise I, Patient 14

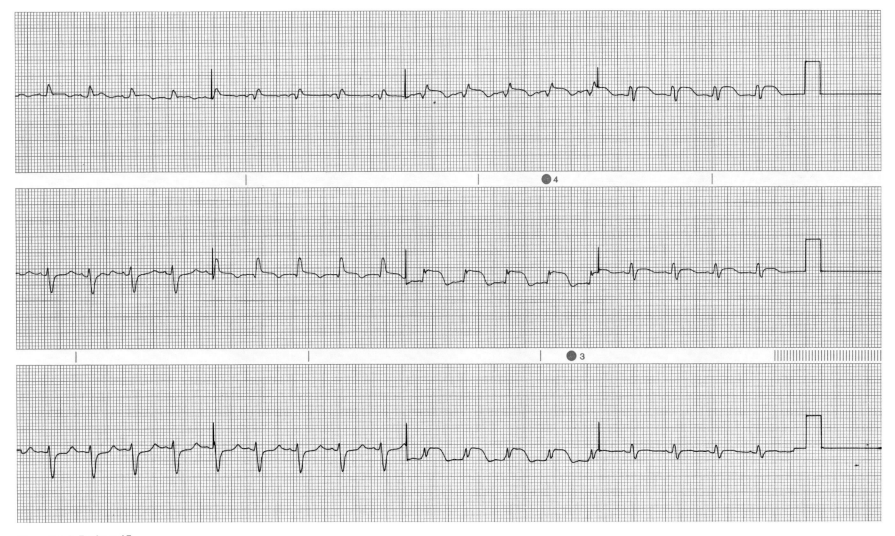

Exercise I, Patient 15

1. This patient shows a normal sinus rhythm. The QRS complex is broad. There is a broad R′ in lead V_1 and a broad terminal S in lead V_6, indicating a right bundle branch block. There is a small Q wave in lead aV_F, which is not broad but could represent an old inferior myocardial infarction. Coded 6, 55, and 86 (and possibly 78 and 94).

2. This patient has a normal sinus rhythm. The PR interval is greater than 200 milliseconds, representing a first-degree atrioventricular (AV) block. There is leftward axis deviation and a nonspecific widening of the QRS complex with secondary ST-T wave changes. The Q in aV_L raises the possibility of an old lateral infarction. This is less certain in view of the nonspecific intraventricular delay. Coded 5, 41, 52, 60, and 86.

3. This patient has a sinus bradycardia. The P wave in lead II is broad and notched. Those in lead V_1 are broadly negative, suggesting left atrial enlargement. There are clear Q waves in leads I, aV_L, and V_6, suggesting an old lateral myocardial infarction, and nonspecific T wave abnormalities in the mid precordial leads. Coded 7, 63, 77, 89, and 94.

4. This patient shows a sinus tachycardia with bursts of supraventricular tachycardia at the end of the first panel, at the beginning of the second panel, and in the fourth panel. The Q waves in the inferior leads are consistent with an old inferior myocardial infarction. There is poor R wave progression (in fact, R wave regression into a Q wave in lead V_3) consistent with an old anterior infarction. The repolarization changes are nonspecific. Coded 6, 22, 76, 78, 89, and 94.

5. This patient has a normal sinus rhythm and right axis deviation. An RSR′ pattern in lead V_1 with the R′ >S and T wave inversion suggests incomplete right bundle branch block and right ventricular hypertrophy. The P waves in lead II and V_1 are tall, suggesting right atrial enlargement. An electrocardiogram like this could be produced by various clinical problems. Right ventricular hypertrophy is indicated, but not necessarily the etiology. Coded 5, 53, 54, 68, and 64.

6. This electrocardiogram shows atrial tachycardia with a variable AV block. The atrial waves are best seen in the third panel. There is a premature ventricular beat terminating the electrocardiogram. There is significant left axis deviation associated with a small Q wave in aV_L, no QRS widening, and T wave inversion, which is consistent with left anterior hemiblock. In the anterior precordial leads, R wave progression is slow with a qrS pattern in lead V_3, consistent with anteroseptal infarction. In leads V_4 and V_5, there are low T waves associated with prominent U waves, consistent with hypokalemia. Coded 13, 23, 58, 75, 93, 98, and 94 (and possibly 101 since atrial tachycardia with block is not infrequently a digitalis toxic rhythm).

7. This electrocardiogram shows a sinus rhythm. The broad notched P wave in lead II is consistent with left atrial enlargement. There is prominent voltage in the lateral leads with slight broadening of the QRS complex and ST and T wave changes in the V_6, which is consistent with left ventricular hypertrophy. Upright, symmetric T waves in the face of left ventricular hypertrophy suggest diastolic overload of the ventricle, which was the case with this patient who had severe mitral insufficiency from mitral valve prolapse. Coded 5, 63, 67, and 86.

8. This is more typical left ventricular hypertrophy with strain. The rhythm is sinus. There is a first-degree AV block. P waves are prominent in lead II and broadly negative in lead V_1, suggesting left atrial enlargement. The increased voltage with a strain pattern seen in lead V_6 is caused by left ventricular hypertrophy. The electrocardiogram has marked left axis deviation, and the QRS duration is < 120 milliseconds, as measured in the three standard limb leads. As a result, this could be called a left anterior hemiblock. Coded 5, 41, 58, 63, 67, and 86.

9. This patient shows negative P waves in leads II and III, suggesting ectopic atrial rhythm. The final beat in panel 1 is broad and different than preceding beats. It is premature, and the compensatory pause suggests premature ventricular contraction. There is left axis deviation, but not great enough to be an anterior hemiblock. There is broadening of the QRS complex to 120 milliseconds, also inconsistent with a diagnosis of anterior hemiblock. The T waves, especially in the lateral precordial leads, are prominent and symmetric, raising the possibility of hyperkalemia. Coded 12, 23, 52, 60, 91, and 97.

10. This patient has an acute infarction. The rhythm is sinus. There is ST segment elevation in the inferior leads as well as V_6. There is a symmetric prominence of the T wave in lead V_5, which is related to this infarct. Reciprocal ST segment depressions are seen in leads aV_L and V_1 to V_4, indicating an acute inferior, and perhaps inferoposterior, infarction. Coded 5, 73, 74, 84, and 94.

11. This patient has a fairly benign-appearing electrocardiogram, although the R wave in lead V_1 is prominent and there is T wave inversion. This might suggest right ventricular hypertrophy, but in view of the short PR interval and delta waves in leads II, III, aV_F, V_3, and V_4, the diagnosis of Wolff-Parkinson-White syndrome (WPW) should be made. Coded 5 and 47 (86 could also be included, although in this case, repolarization, except for that in lead V_1, is unremarkable).

12. This patient has a sinus rhythm. There is left axis deviation with a small Q wave and minimal delay in depolarization in lead aV_L, consistent with anterior hemiblock. There are Q

waves in leads V_1 to V_4 caused by anteroseptal infarction. There is a premature ventricular beat with postectopic delay and intermittent, appropriate firing of a ventricular pacemaker. Coded 5, 23, 35, 37, 58, 75, and 94.

13. This patient has an atrial pacemaker with a fixed rate and complete control of the electrocardiogram. There are Q waves in leads II, III, aV_F, and V_6 and T wave changes with slight ST segment elevation suggesting myocardial infarction of uncertain age. Coded 34, 36, 78, and 94.

14. This is an irregularly irregular rhythm of atrial fibrillation. There is ST segment depression in the lateral leads with a relatively short QT interval, which is consistent with digitalis effect. Prominent voltage in the lateral leads raises the possibility of ventricular hypertrophy. Coded 14 and 88 (and possibly 66).

15. This is another patient with coronary artery disease. There is sinus tachycardia and left axis deviation with a small Q wave and repolarization changes in lead aV_L, suggesting anterior hemiblock. In the precordial leads there is marked ST segment elevation in leads V_1 to V_4 with slight elevation in leads V_5 and aV_L, all consistent with an acute anterior infarct. There is a terminal positive QRS vector in lead V_1, suggesting incomplete right bundle branch block. Coded 6, 54, 58, 70, 84, and 94 (and possibly 72).

Exercise II

ANSWER SHEET
Exercise II

Patient 1 ___ ___ ___ ___ ___ ___ ___ ___

Patient 2 ___ ___ ___ ___ ___ ___ ___ ___

Patient 3 ___ ___ ___ ___ ___ ___ ___ ___

Patient 4 ___ ___ ___ ___ ___ ___ ___ ___

Patient 5 ___ ___ ___ ___ ___ ___ ___ ___

Patient 6 ___ ___ ___ ___ ___ ___ ___ ___

Patient 7 ___ ___ ___ ___ ___ ___ ___ ___

Patient 8 ___ ___ ___ ___ ___ ___ ___ ___

Patient 9 ___ ___ ___ ___ ___ ___ ___ ___

Patient 10 ___ ___ ___ ___ ___ ___ ___ ___

Patient 11 ___ ___ ___ ___ ___ ___ ___ ___

Patient 12 ___ ___ ___ ___ ___ ___ ___ ___

Patient 13 ___ ___ ___ ___ ___ ___ ___ ___

Patient 14 ___ ___ ___ ___ ___ ___ ___ ___

Patient 15 ___ ___ ___ ___ ___ ___ ___ ___

Electrocardiographic Diagnostic Coding Sheet

General Features
1. Normal ECG
2. Normal ECG, variant
3. Misplaced leads
4. Electrical alternans

Sinus Rhythms
5. Normal sinus
6. Sinus tachycardia
7. Sinus bradycardia
8. Sinus arrhythmia
9. Sinus pause or arrest

Atrial Rhythms
10. Premature atrial contractions (PAC)
11. Aberrant PAC
12. Ectopic atrial rhythm
13. Atrial tachycardia with AV block
14. Atrial fibrillation
15. Atrial flutter
16. Multifocal atrial tachycardia
17. Dual atrial rhythms

AV Junctional Rhythms
18. Premature junctional beats (PJB)
19. Aberrant PJB
20. Junctional beat or rhythm
21. AV junctional rhythm with retrograde atrial activation
22. Supraventricular tachycardia

Ventricular Rhythms
23. Premature ventricular contractions (PVC), unifocal
24. PVC, multifocal
25. PVC, couplets/triplets
26. PVC, R-on-T
27. Ventricular tachycardia
28. Idioventricular rhythm
29. Ventricular fibrillation
30. Ventricular escape beat or rhythm
31. Ventricular fusion beat or rhythm
32. Ventricular capture beat during VT
33. Torsades de pointes

Pacemaker Rhythms
34. Fixed rate
35. Demand
36. Atrial pacing
37. Ventricular pacing
38. Dual chamber pacing
39. Failure to sense
40. Failure to capture

AV Conduction Abnormalities
41. 1° AV block
42. Wenckebach (Mobitz I) AV block
43. 2° AV block (Mobitz II)
44. Fixed 2° AV block, 2:1, 4:1, etc.
45. Complete heart block
46. Variable AV block
47. Preexcitation (WPW)

AV - VA Interactions
48. Fusion beat
49. Echo beat
50. AV dissociation
51. Isorhythmic AV dissociation

Intraventricular Conduction Abnormalities
52. Left axis
53. Right axis
54. Incomplete RBBB
55. Complete RBBB
56. Incomplete LBBB
57. Complete LBBB
58. Anterior hemiblock
59. Posterior hemiblock
60. Nonspecific IVCD
61. Arrhythmia related aberrancy
62. Intermittent IVCD/BBB

Chamber Enlargement
63. Left atrial enlargement
64. Right atrial enlargement
65. Bi-atrial enlargement
66. LVH - voltage
67. LVH - voltage plus repolarization changes
68. RVH
69. Biventricular hypertrophy

Myocardial Infarction

Recent/Acute
70. Anteroseptal
71. Anterior
72. Lateral
73. Inferior
74. Posterior

Old/Uncertain Age
75. Anteroseptal
76. Anterior
77. Lateral
78. Inferior
79. Posterior

Repolarization Changes
80. Possible LV aneurysm
81. Non-Q wave infarction
82. Early repolarization
83. Persistent juvenile T wave
84. ST-T wave changes of acute injury
85. ST-T wave changes of acute ischemia
86. ST-T wave changes of hypertrophy or altered intraventricular conduction (secondary repolarization changes)
87. ST-T wave changes of pericarditis
88. ST changes due to digitalis effect
89. Nonspecific ST-T wave changes
90. Postectopic T wave changes
91. Peaked T waves
92. Prolonged QT interval
93. Prominent U waves

Clinical Problems
94. Coronary artery disease
95. Congenital heart disease
96. Mitral valve disease
97. Hyperkalemia
98. Hypokalemia
99. Hypercalcemia
100. Hypocalcemia
101. Digitalis toxicity
102. CNS event
103. Motion artifact
104. Dextrocardia
105. Cardiac tamponade
106. Cardiac transplant
107. Chronic lung disease

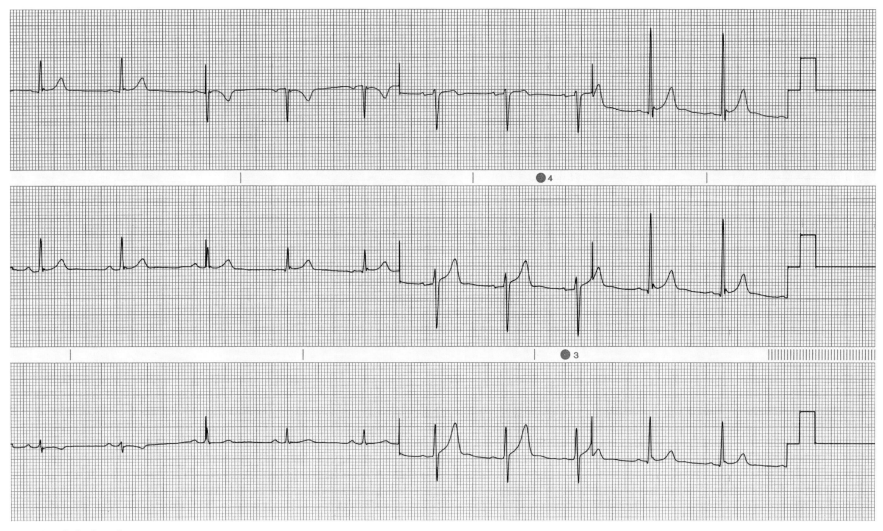

Exercise II, Patient 1

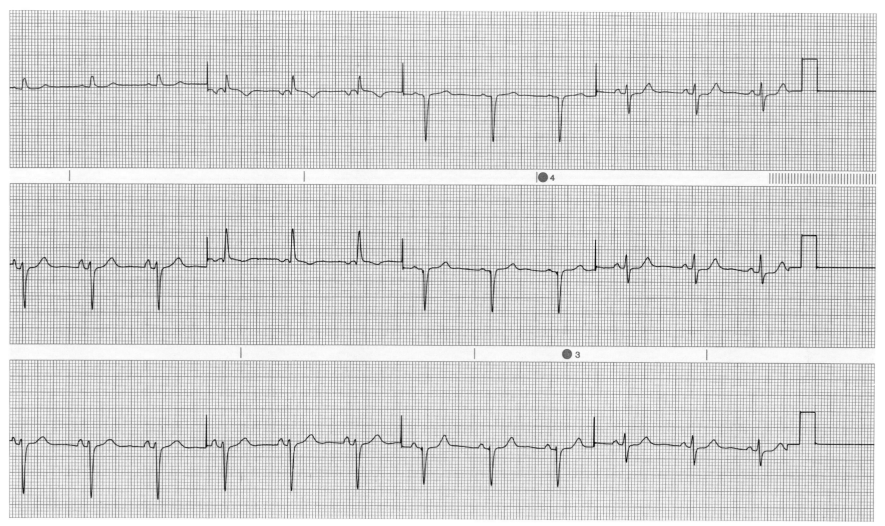

Exercise II, Patient 2

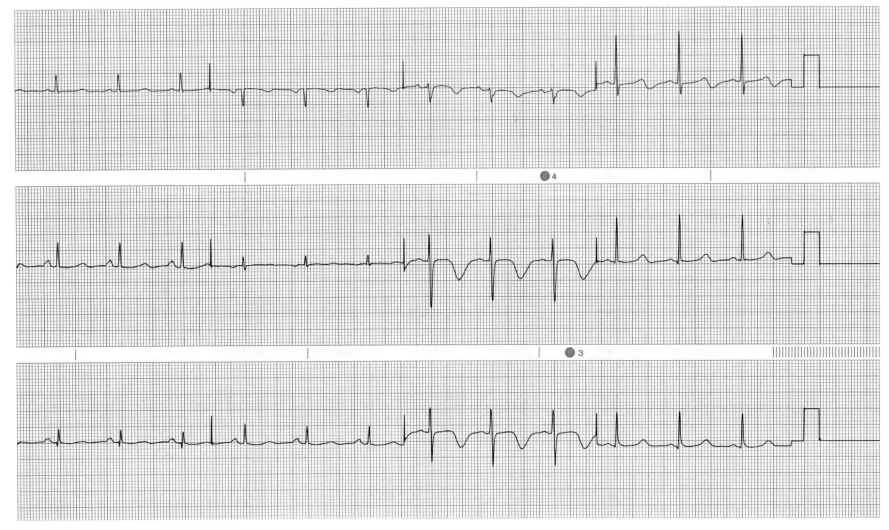

Exercise II, Patient 3

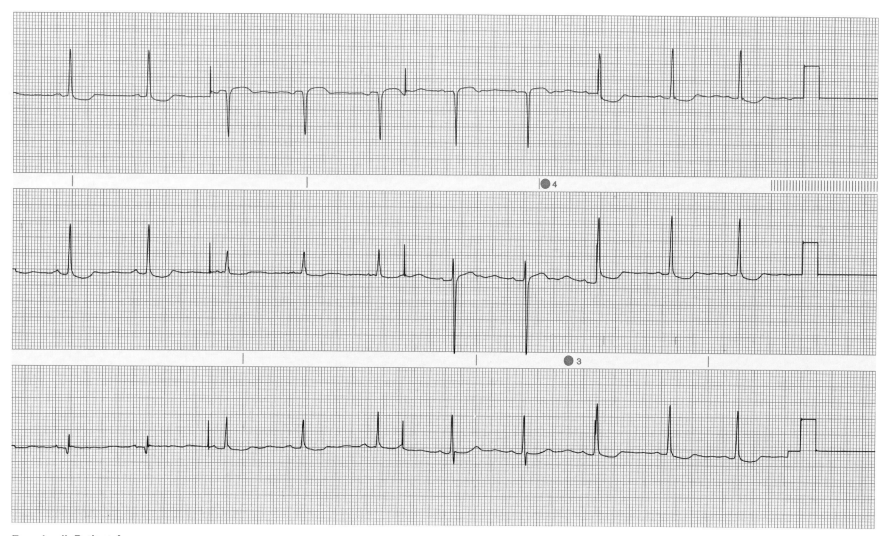

Exercise II, Patient 4

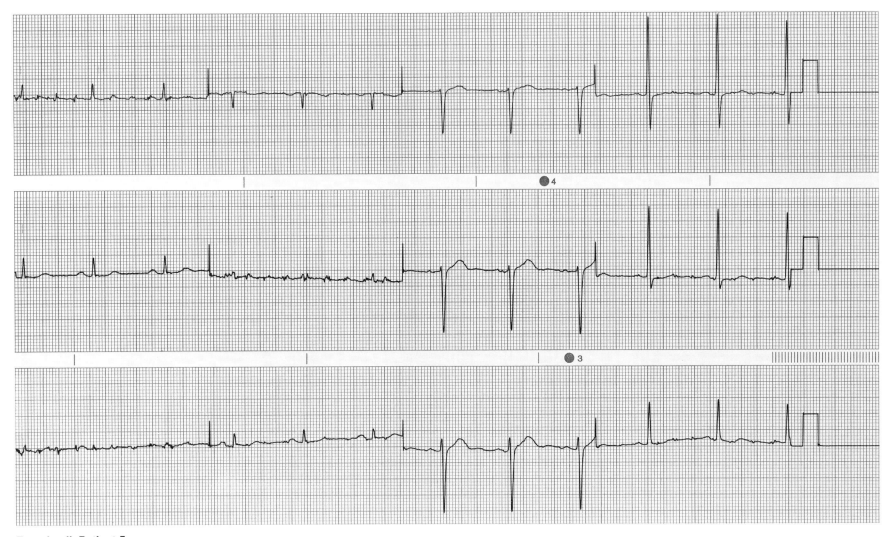

Exercise II, Patient 5

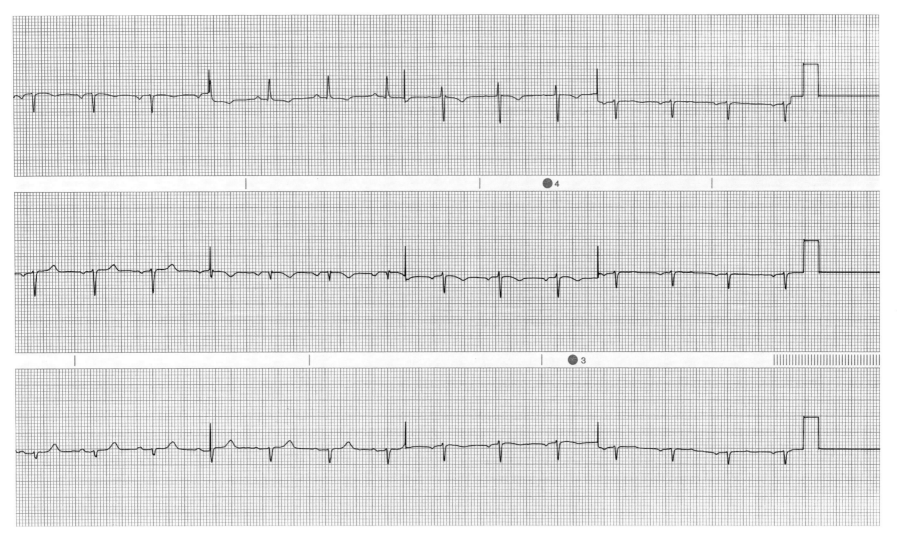

Exercise II, Patient 6

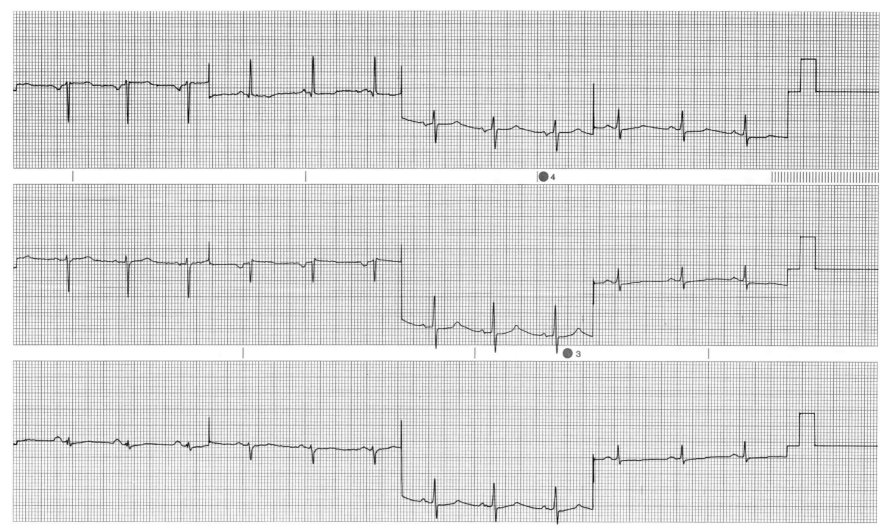

Exercise II, Patient 7

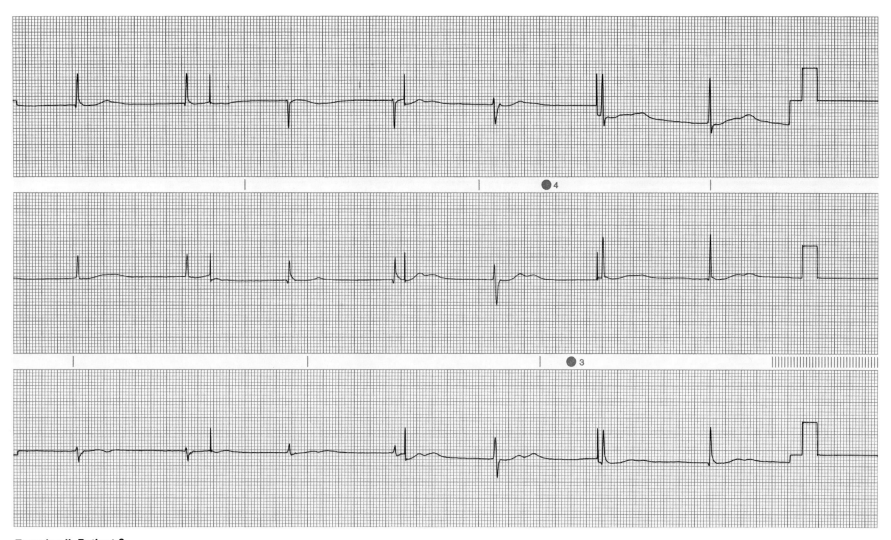

Exercise II, Patient 8

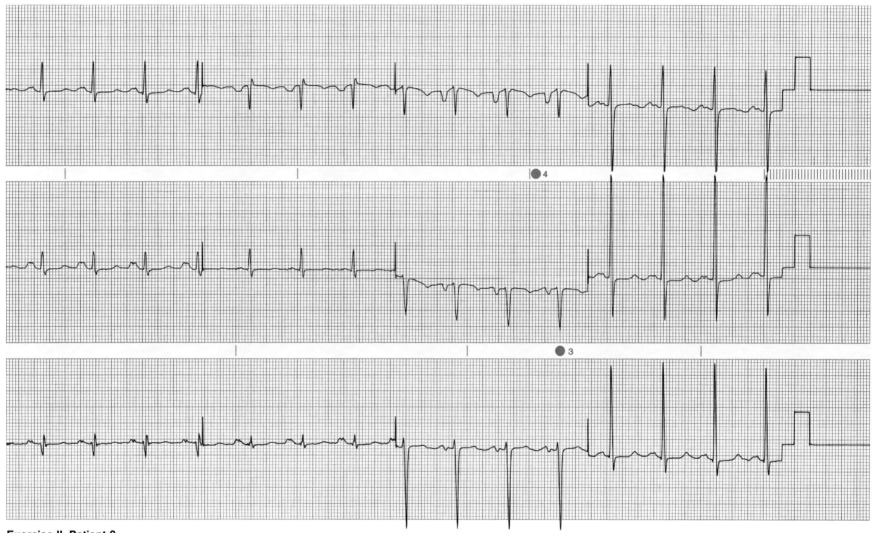

Exercise II, Patient 9

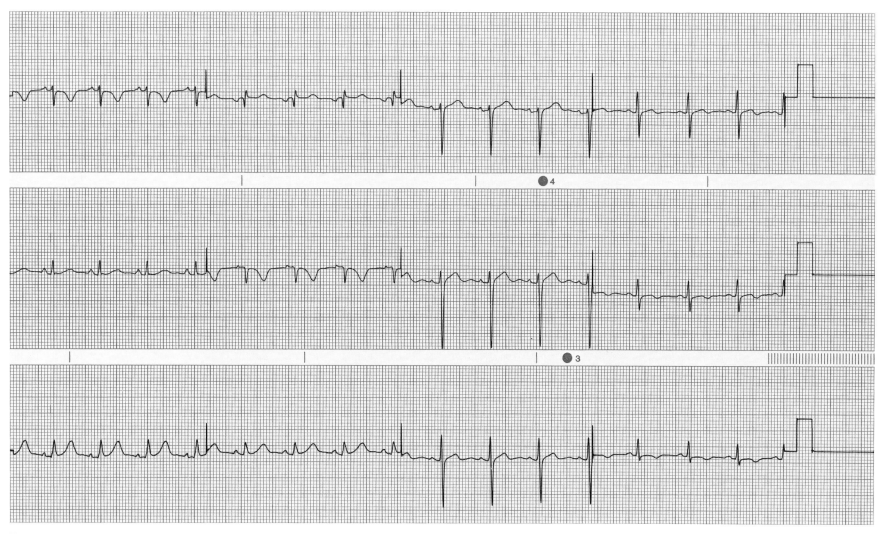

Exercise II, Patient 10

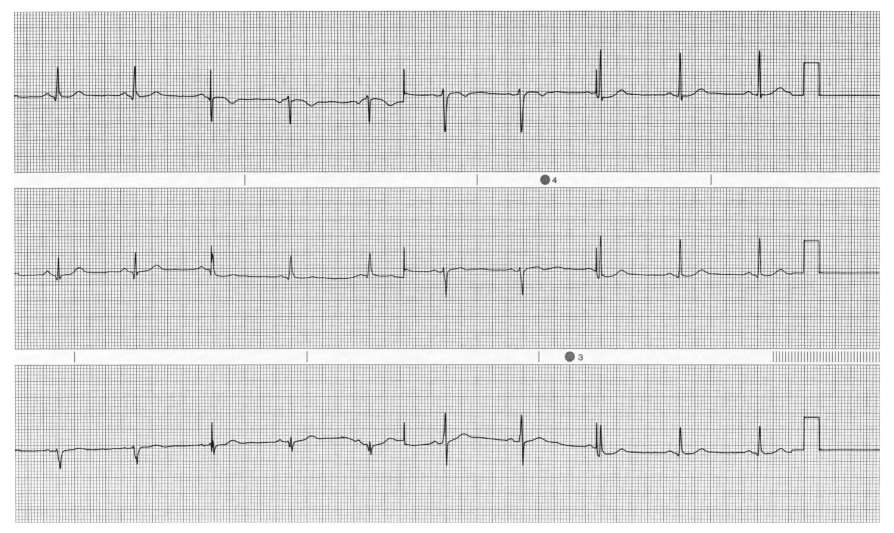

Exercise II, Patient 11

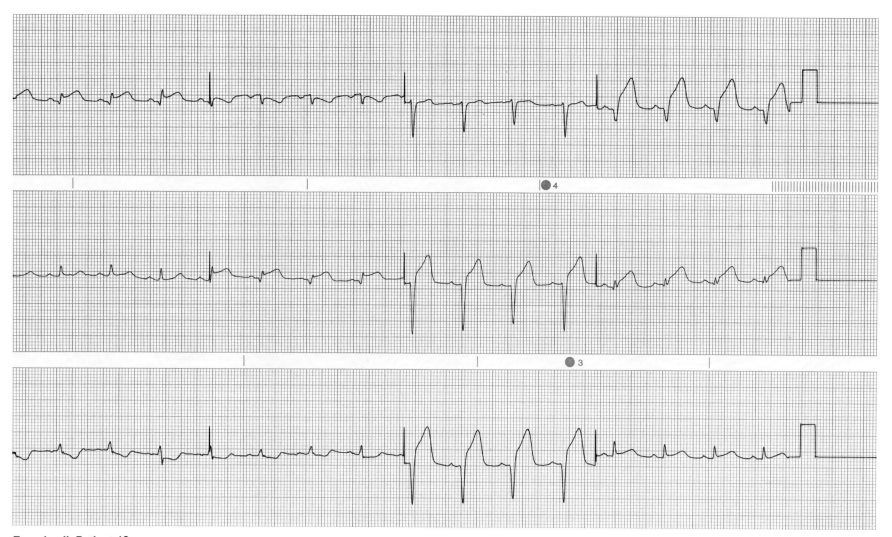

Exercise II, Patient 12

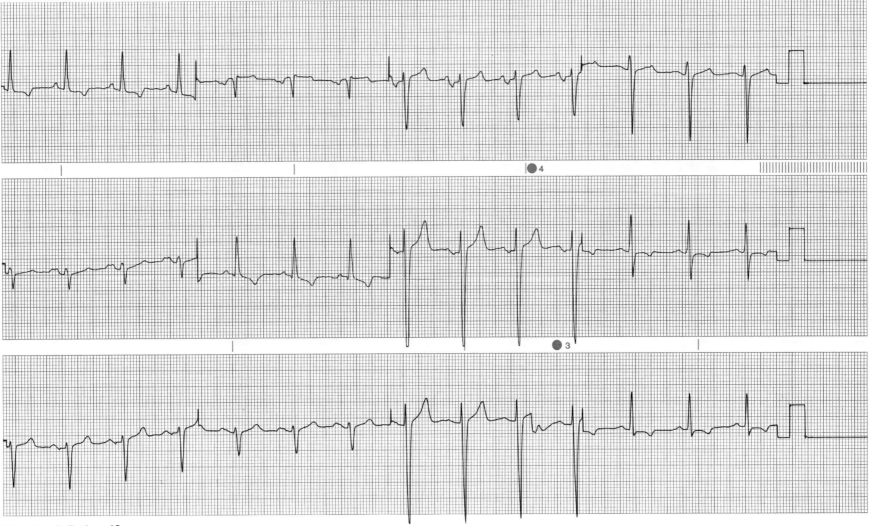

Exercise II, Patient 13

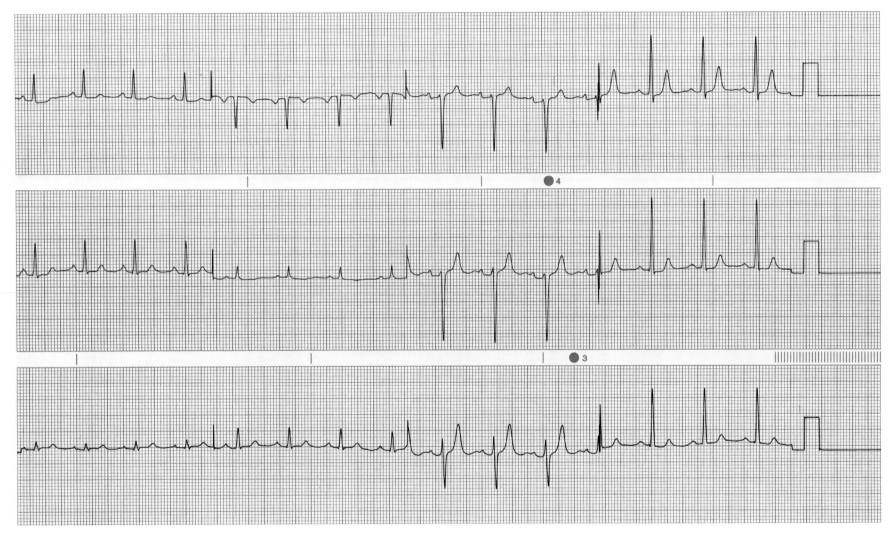

Exercise II, Patient 14

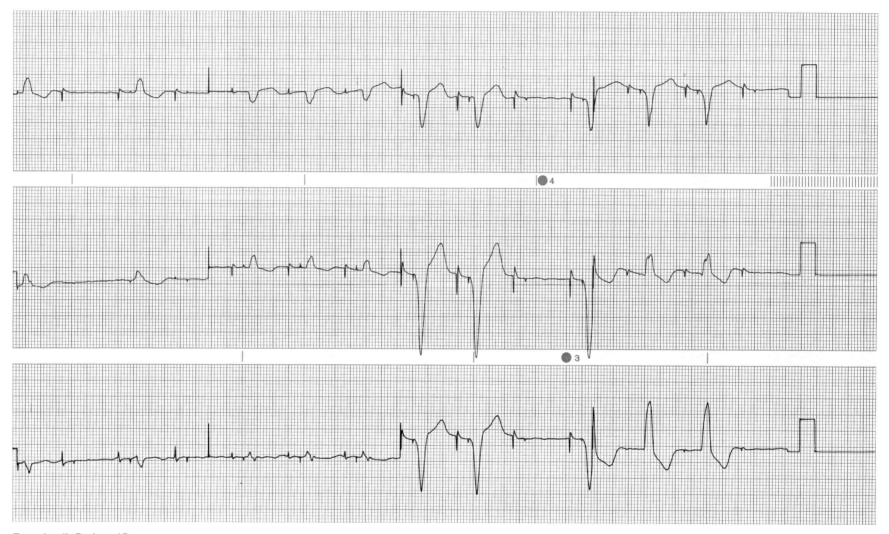

Exercise II, Patient 15

1. This patient shows a sinus rhythm with ST segment elevation in the mid precordial leads. T waves, however, are normal and the electrocardiogram is otherwise unremarkable. This is an example of early repolarization, which is a normal variant. Coded 2, 5, and 82.

2. This patient has a sinus rhythm and marked left axis deviation. In lead aV_L there is a small Q wave, delay in repolarization, and secondary repolarization changes. The axis and changes in aV_L are consistent with an anterior hemiblock. In the third panel, there are Q waves in leads V_1 to V_3, suggesting anteroseptal myocardial infarction. Repolarization is normal; this is an old infarct. Coded 5, 58, 75, and 94.

3. This patient has a sinus rhythm. The most notable abnormality is a broad QT interval with symmetric T wave inversion in the mid precordial leads. T wave changes like this can be seen chronically with non-Q wave infarctions, but in this case, the symmetric and very broad quality suggests a recent CNS event, which was the case in this patient. Coded 5, 92, and 102.

4. This patient has a sinus rhythm. ST segments are depressed and scooped with the QT interval relatively short, suggesting digitalis effect. Coded 5 and 88.

5. This patient has a sinus rhythm that is most clearly seen in leads V_1 and V_2. In the limb leads there is a regular distortion of the baseline caused by a somatic tremor. In the lateral precordial leads there is reduced amplitude of T waves, a nonspecific finding. Coded 5, 89, and 103. Parkinson's disease would come to mind in a tracing like this.

6. This is an abnormal electrocardiogram. The P waves in leads I and II are inverted. There is a drop-off in voltage across the precordium. This combination is seen with dextrocardia. Coded 5 and 104.

7. This electrocardiogram also shows negative P waves in lead I and an abnormal P vector in lead II. Unlike the preceding electrocardiogram, the R wave evolution is normal, although there are some nonspecific ST-T wave changes laterally. This is consistent with switched arm leads, a technical error. Coded 3, 5, and 89.

8. This electrocardiogram shows a slow rate that is subtly irregular and represents slow atrial fibrillation. In the lateral precordial leads the T waves are low and broad and are associated with prominent U waves, raising the possibility of hypokalemia. Coded 14, 93, and 98.

9. This patient has a sinus rhythm. The P waves are broad and notched in lead II and broadly negative in lead V_1. The voltages are prominent in the lateral precordial leads, and there are T wave abnormalities. This would be consistent with left atrial enlargement and left ventricular hypertrophy. Coded 5, 63, and 66.

10. This patient has a sinus rhythm. There are repolarization changes in the lateral precordial leads, which are abnormal but nonspecific. The T wave inversion in leads I and aV_L and the Q wave in aV_L raise the possibility of old high lateral myocardial infarction. Coded 5, 77, 89, and 94.

11. This is a normal electrocardiogram. The rhythm is sinus. T waves evolve in a normal fashion, as do the R waves. All of the intervals are within normal limits. Coded 1.

12. This patient has coronary disease. Rhythm is sinus. ST segment elevation in the anterior and lateral leads is consistent with an acute infarction. ST depression in leads aV_F and III supports that diagnosis. Coded 5, 71, 72, 84, and 94.

13. This patient has sinus rhythm. T wave and ST segment changes in the lateral precordial and lateral limb leads with high voltage suggest left ventricular hypertrophy. The P waves are broad and notched in lead II, and there is a prominent, negative, terminal vector of the P wave in V_1, suggesting left atrial enlargement. Coded 5, 52, 63, 67, and 86.

14. This patient has a sinus rhythm. The T waves in the mid precordial leads are narrow and prominent, raising the possibility of hyperkalemia. Coded 5, 91, and 97.

15. This electrocardiogram shows AV sequential, or at least dual-chamber, pacing. The rate is fixed, but there is intermittent failure to capture. Coded 38 and 40.

Exercise III

ANSWER SHEET
Exercise III

Patient 1 —— —— —— —— —— —— —— ——

Patient 2 —— —— —— —— —— —— —— ——

Patient 3 —— —— —— —— —— —— —— ——

Patient 4 —— —— —— —— —— —— —— ——

Patient 5 —— —— —— —— —— —— —— ——

Patient 6 —— —— —— —— —— —— —— ——

Patient 7 —— —— —— —— —— —— —— ——

Patient 8 —— —— —— —— —— —— —— ——

Patient 9 —— —— —— —— —— —— —— ——

Patient 10 —— —— —— —— —— —— —— ——

Patient 11 —— —— —— —— —— —— —— ——

Patient 12 —— —— —— —— —— —— —— ——

Patient 13 —— —— —— —— —— —— —— ——

Patient 14 —— —— —— —— —— —— —— ——

Patient 15 —— —— —— —— —— —— —— ——

Electrocardiographic Diagnostic Coding Sheet

General Features
1. Normal ECG
2. Normal ECG, variant
3. Misplaced leads
4. Electrical alternans

Sinus Rhythms
5. Normal sinus
6. Sinus tachycardia
7. Sinus bradycardia
8. Sinus arrhythmia
9. Sinus pause or arrest

Atrial Rhythms
10. Premature atrial contractions (PAC)
11. Aberrant PAC
12. Ectopic atrial rhythm
13. Atrial tachycardia with AV block
14. Atrial fibrillation
15. Atrial flutter
16. Multifocal atrial tachycardia
17. Dual atrial rhythms

AV Junctional Rhythms
18. Premature junctional beats (PJB)
19. Aberrant PJB
20. Junctional beat or rhythm
21. AV junctional rhythm with retrograde atrial activation
22. Supraventricular tachycardia

Ventricular Rhythms
23. Premature ventricular contractions (PVC), unifocal
24. PVC, multifocal
25. PVC, couplets/triplets
26. PVC, R-on-T phenomenon
27. Ventricular tachycardia
28. Idioventricular rhythm
29. Ventricular fibrillation
30. Ventricular escape beat or rhythm
31. Ventricular fusion beat or rhythm
32. Ventricular capture beat during VT
33. Torsades de pointes

Pacemaker Rhythms
34. Fixed rate
35. Demand
36. Atrial pacing
37. Ventricular pacing
38. Dual chamber pacing
39. Failure to sense
40. Failure to capture

AV Conduction Abnormalities
41. 1° AV block
42. Wenckebach (Mobitz I) AV block
43. 2° AV block (Mobitz II)
44. Fixed 2° AV block, 2:1, 4:1, etc.
45. Complete heart block
46. Variable AV block
47. Preexcitation (WPW)

AV - VA Interactions
48. Fusion beat
49. Echo beat
50. AV dissociation
51. Isorhythmic AV dissociation

Intraventricular Conduction Abnormalities
52. Left axis
53. Right axis
54. Incomplete RBBB
55. Complete RBBB
56. Incomplete LBBB
57. Complete LBBB
58. Anterior hemiblock
59. Posterior hemiblock
60. Nonspecific IVCD
61. Arrhythmia related aberrancy
62. Intermittent IVCD/BBB

Chamber Enlargement
63. Left atrial enlargement
64. Right atrial enlargement
65. Bi-atrial enlargement
66. LVH - voltage
67. LVH - voltage plus repolarization changes
68. RVH
69. Biventricular hypertrophy

Myocardial Infarction

Recent/Acute
70. Anteroseptal
71. Anterior
72. Lateral
73. Inferior
74. Posterior

Old/Uncertain Age
75. Anteroseptal
76. Anterior
77. Lateral
78. Inferior
79. Posterior

Repolarization Changes
80. Possible LV aneurysm
81. Non-Q wave infarction
82. Early repolarization
83. Persistent juvenile T wave
84. ST-T wave changes of acute injury
85. ST-T wave changes of acute ischemia
86. ST-T wave changes of hypertrophy or altered intraventricular conduction (secondary repolarization changes)
87. ST-T wave changes of pericarditis
88. ST changes due to digitalis effect
89. Nonspecific ST-T wave changes
90. Postectopic T wave changes
91. Peaked T waves
92. Prolonged QT interval
93. Prominent U waves

Clinical Problems
94. Coronary artery disease
95. Congenital heart disease
96. Mitral valve disease
97. Hyperkalemia
98. Hypokalemia
99. Hypercalcemia
100. Hypocalcemia
101. Digitalis toxicity
102. CNS event
103. Motion artifact
104. Dextrocardia
105. Cardiac tamponade
106. Cardiac transplant
107. Chronic lung disease

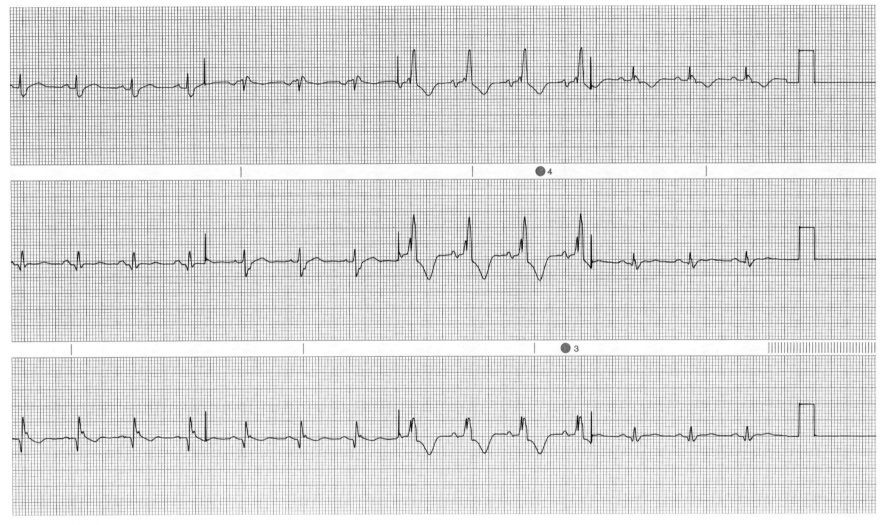

Exercise III, Patient 1

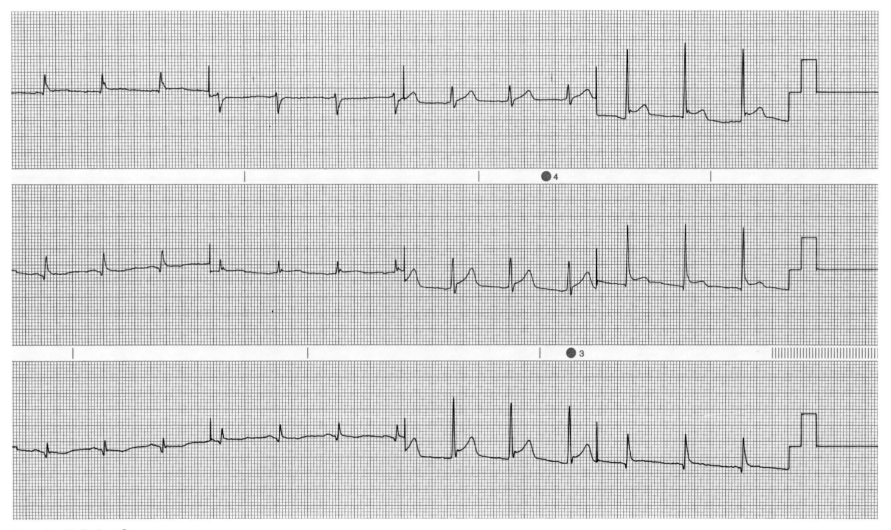

Exercise III, Patient 2

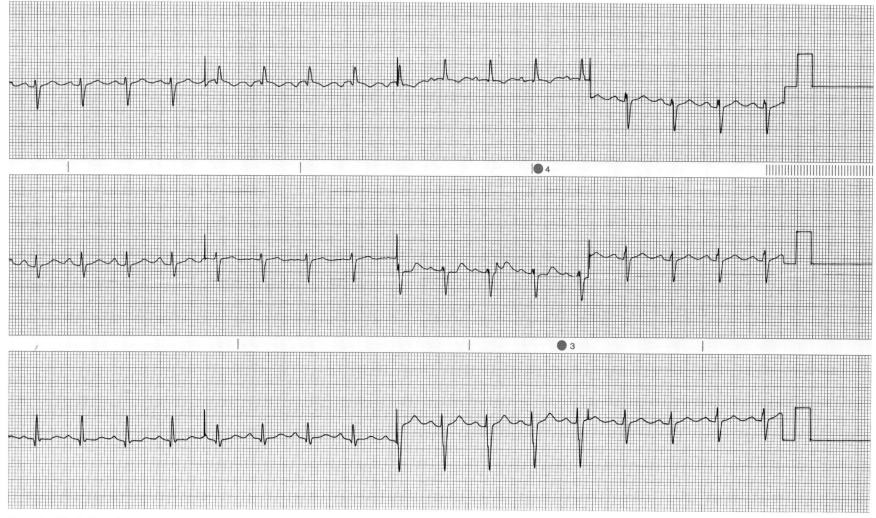

Exercise III, Patient 3

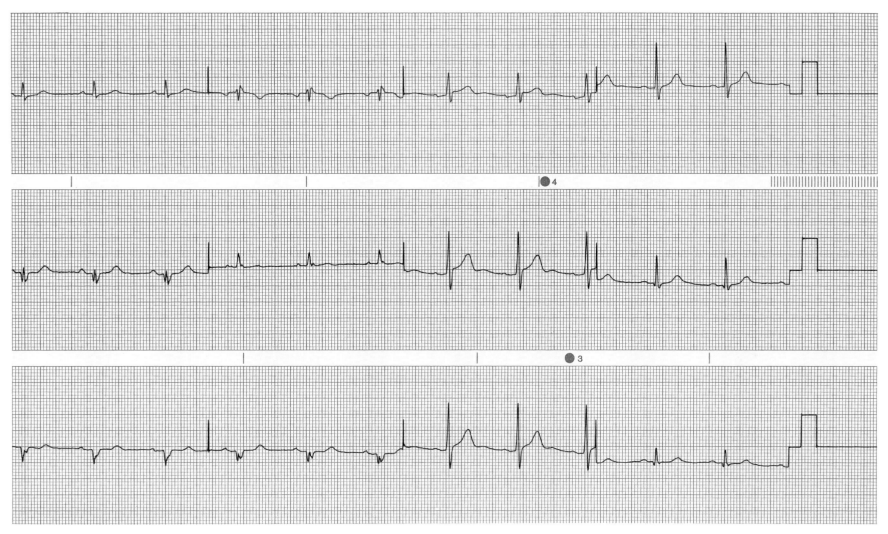

Exercise III, Patient 4

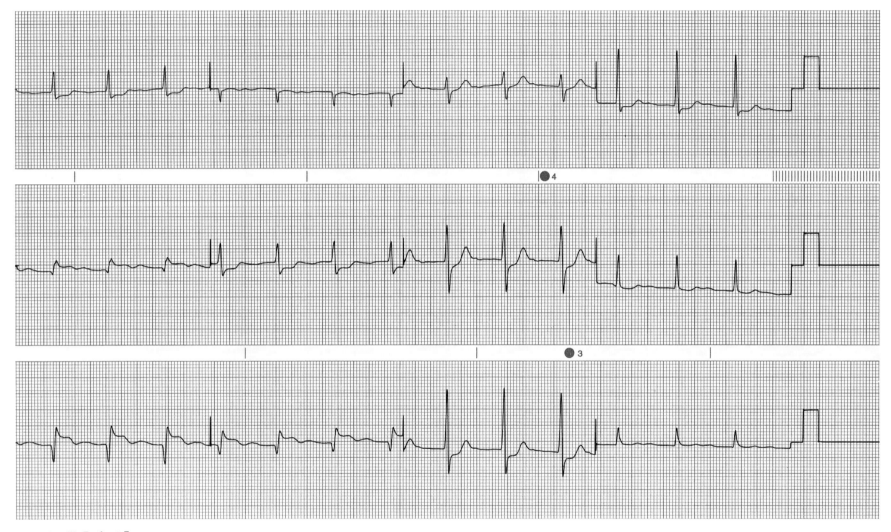

Exercise III, Patient 5

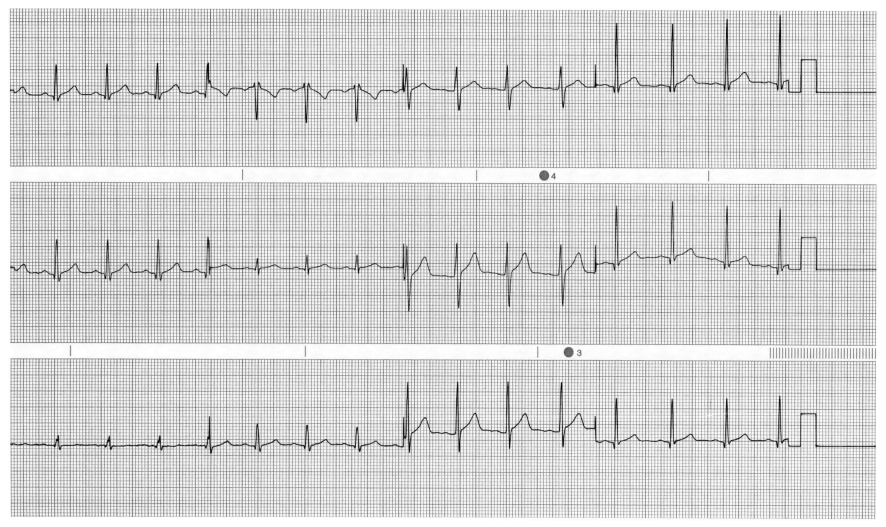

Exercise III, Patient 6

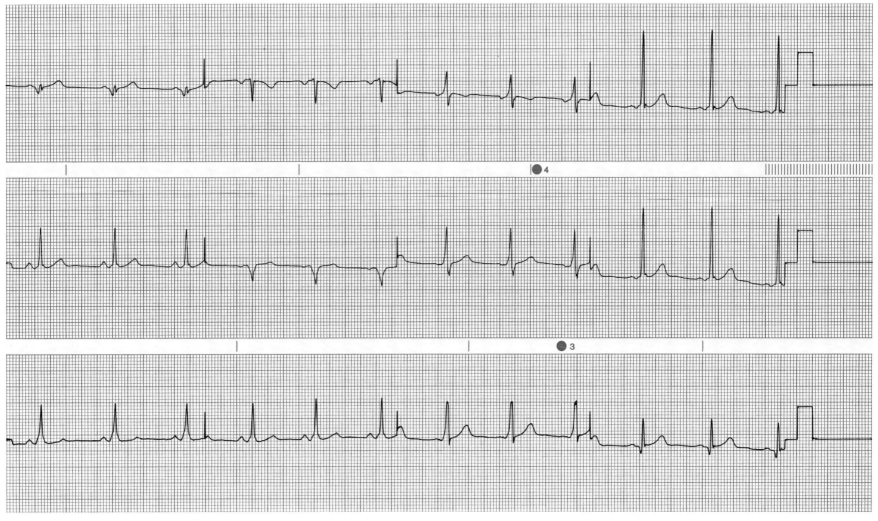

Exercise III, Patient 7

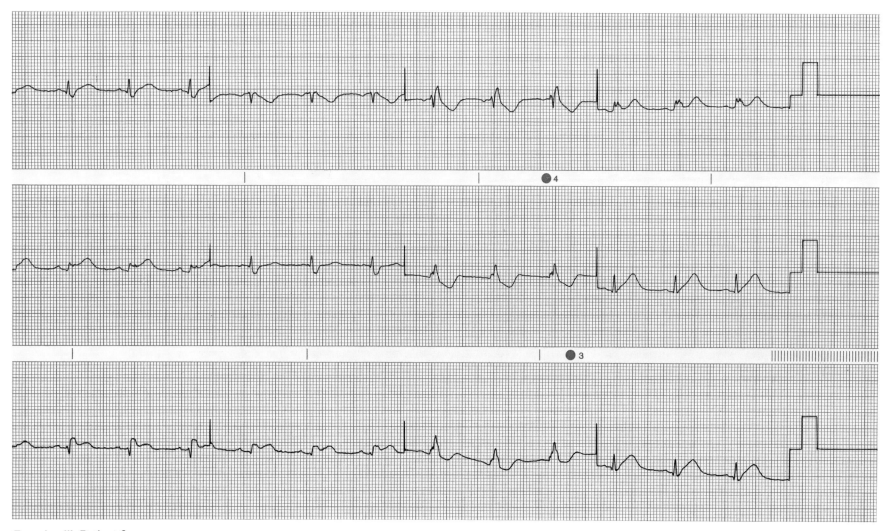

Exercise III, Patient 8

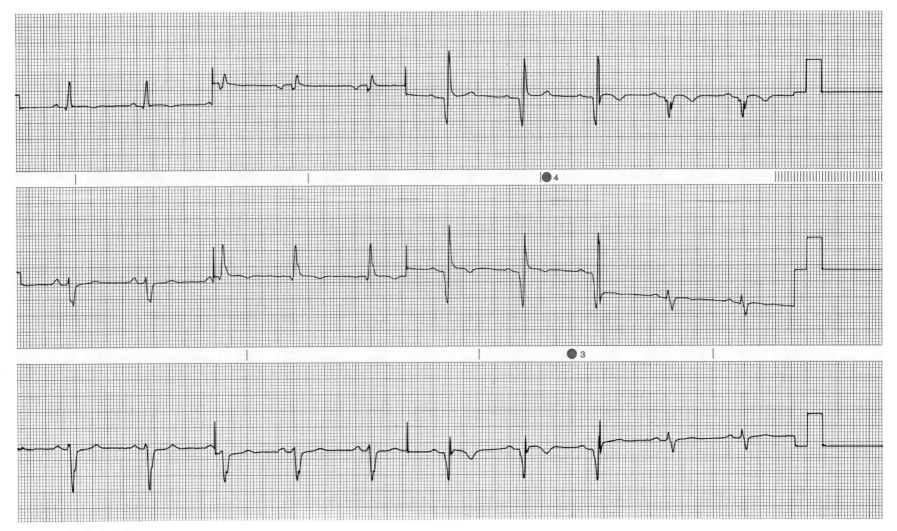

Exercise III, Patient 9

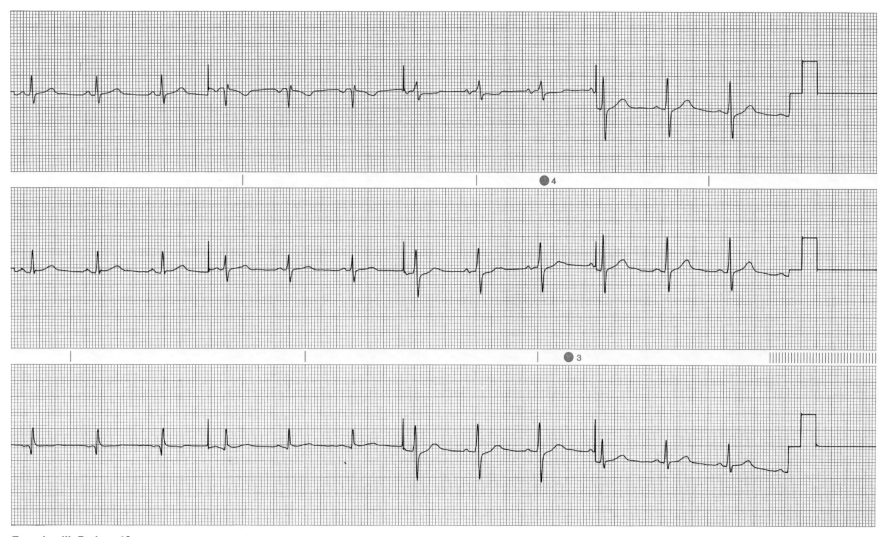

Exercise III, Patient 10

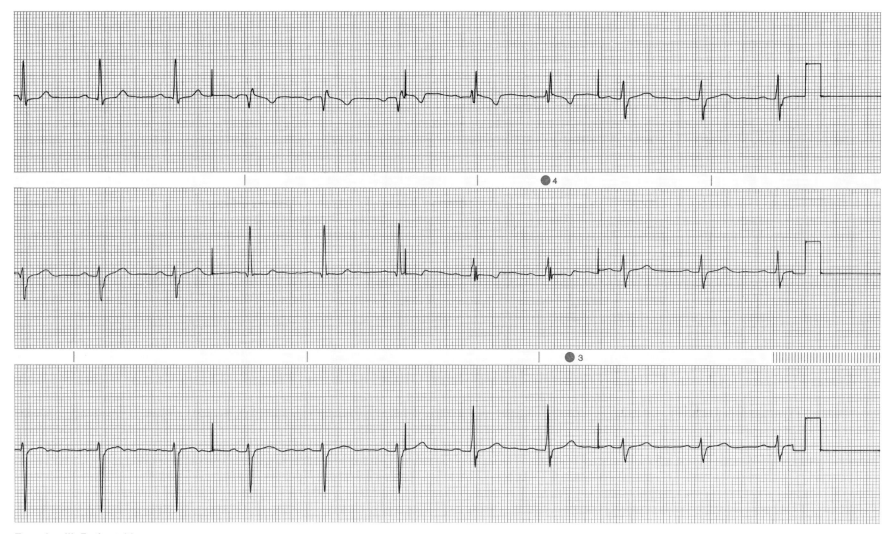

Exercise III, Patient 11

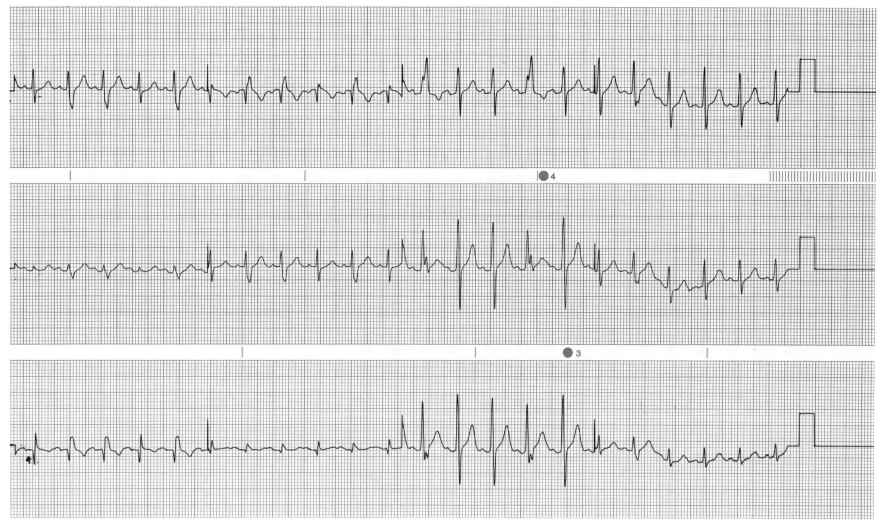

Exercise III, Patient 12

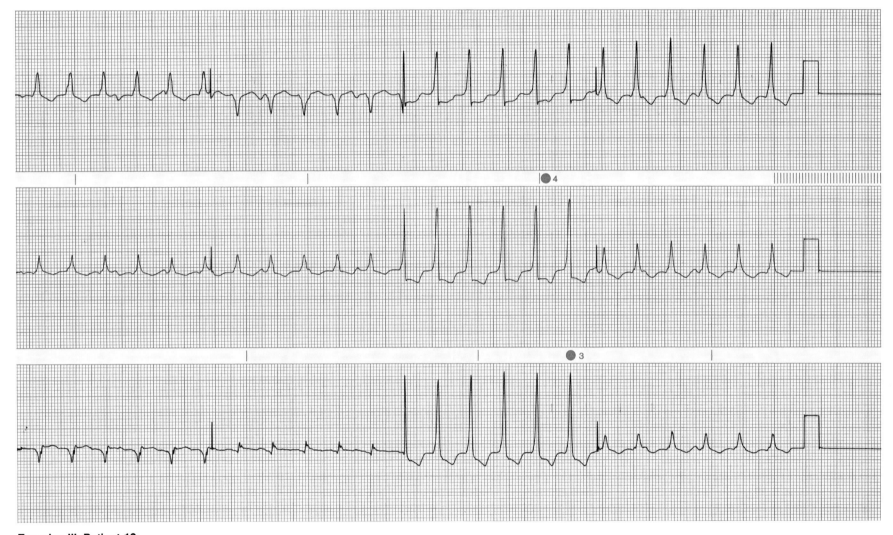

Exercise III, Patient 13

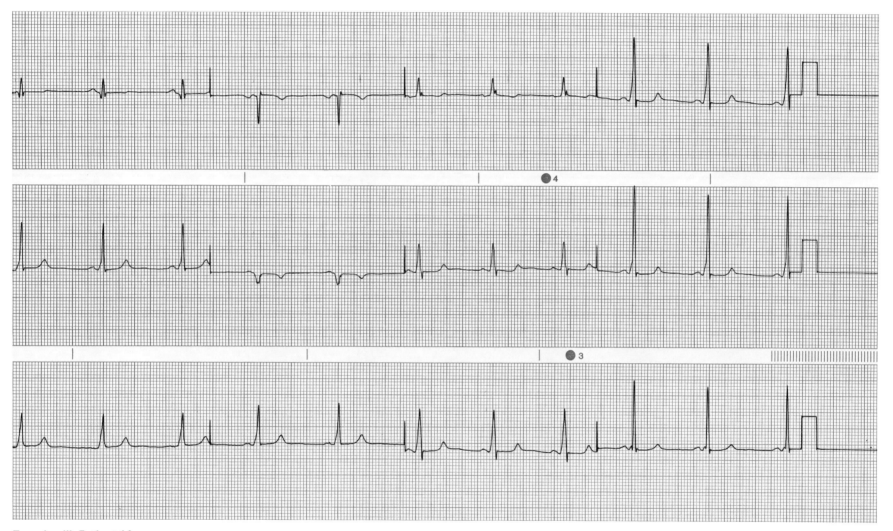

Exercise III, Patient 14

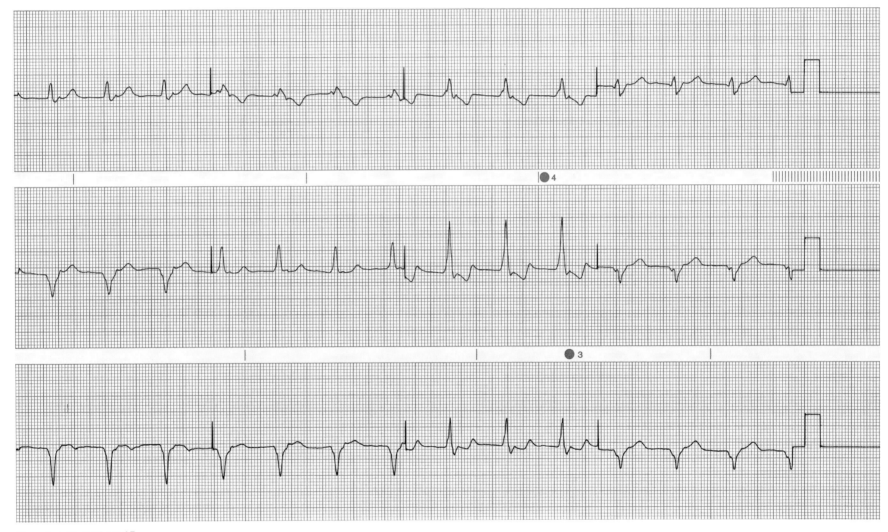

Exercise III, Patient 15

1. This patient has a sinus rhythm. There are significant Q waves in leads II, III, and aV_F. There are also Q waves in lead V_5 and especially in lead V_6. Lead V_1 shows broadening of the QRS with a broad R', and in lead V_6 a broad terminal S is consistent with right bundle branch block. This is a right bundle branch block with inferior and lateral myocardial infarctions, both old. Coded 5, 55, 77, 78, and 94.

2. This patient has a sinus rhythm. There are significant Q waves in lead aV_F and prominent, dominant R waves in leads V_1 and V_2 with an upright T wave, consistent with inferoposterior infarction. There is generalized ST segment elevation from pericarditis rather than an acute infarct. Coded 5, 78, 79, 87, and 94.

3. This electrocardiogram also shows prominent R waves in lead V_1. There is T wave inversion in lead V_1 and right axis deviation, indicating right ventricular hypertrophy. This young woman had obliterative pulmonary vascular disease caused by a mixed connective tissue syndrome leading to pulmonary hypertension and right ventricular hypertrophy. Coded 6, 53, and 68.

4. This is another inferoposterior infarct. There are broad Q waves in leads II, III, and aV_F. The R wave is greater than S in lead V_1, and the T wave is upright. Coded 5, 78, 79, and 94.

5. This is an acute inferior infarct with probably some posterior involvement. There is acute ST segment elevation with the beginning of T wave inversion in the inferior leads. ST segment depression is present in lead I and aV_L. Q waves have begun to emerge in leads aV_F, III, and to some extent, II. This is an acute or recent infarct. The rhythm is sinus with first-degree AV block. Coded 5, 41, 73, 84, and 94.

6. This patient has a sinus rhythm and prominence of the R wave in lead V_1. There really are no other abnormalities on this electrocardiogram. This could be a pure posterior infarct or an example of marked counterclockwise rotation, a normal variant. In fact, this 27-year-old man had no risk factors or symptoms of coronary disease. Coded 2 and 5. (An old pure posterior infarct diagnosed on this electrocardiogram, would not be incorrect; coded 79 and 94.)

7. This electrocardiogram also shows prominence of the R wave forces in lead V_1. There is T wave inversion, which is consistent with right ventricular hypertrophy. However, delta waves are clearly seen in many leads, and the PR interval is short. This is an example of a sinus rhythm with Wolff-Parkinson-White syndrome and a pseudo right ventricular hypertrophy pattern. Coded 5 and 47.

8. This patient has a sinus rhythm. The QRS is greater than 120 milliseconds with a prominent broad R' in lead V_1 and a broad terminal S in lead V_6. This is a right bundle branch block. In the inferior leads there is acute ST segment elevation and symmetric T wave prominence in leads V_5 and V_6. This is suggestive of acute inferior infarction with hyperacute T waves in the lateral leads. Coded 5, 55, 73, 84, and 94.

9. This patient has a sinus rhythm, a right bundle branch block, anterior hemiblock, and an anteroseptal infarction. The PR interval is normal. The QRS, however, is broad. The terminal vector in lead V_1 is positive and wide. There is a broad terminal S in lead V_6, indicating a right bundle branch block. There is marked left axis deviation and a small Q and aV_L consistent with anterior hemiblock. The septal and anterior forces have been removed by anterior and septal in-

farction, producing the QR pattern in leads V_1 to V_3 and a pure Q in lead V_4. Coded 5, 55, 58, 75, and 94.

10. This is a pure posterior infarct, with R > S in lead V_1 and upright T waves in that lead. There is a Q in lead III, with no other abnormalities. As with patient 6 in this exercise, this could be a normal variant and an example of marked counterclockwise rotation of the heart. But in this case the patient had coronary disease. Coded 5, 79, and 94.

11. This patient has a sinus rhythm. There is a prominent R' in lead V_1 with T wave inversion. The QRS complex is not broad and represents an incomplete (not complete) right bundle branch block. An incomplete right bundle with an R' > S indicates right ventricular hypertrophy. This case is unusual in that the axis is leftward. This raises the possibility of congenital heart disease with an ostium primum atrial septal defect (ASD). This degree of left axis ordinarily would suggest anterior hemiblock, but in the face of an ostium primum ASD, a simple call of left axis deviation probably is more correct. Coded 5, 41, 52, 54, 68, and 95.

12. This patient has a sinus rhythm. There is intermittent right bundle branch block, which can be seen in all the panels. In the beats that do not conduct with the right bundle branch block pattern, the R wave is prominent in lead V_1, the T wave is upright, and there are small inferior Q waves, suggesting there is also an old posterior (perhaps inferoposterior) myocardial infarction. Coded 6, 62, 79, and 94 (and possibly 78).

13. This patient has a wide complex tachycardia with prominent R waves in lead V_1. The underlying rhythm is sinus, as can be seen in the first panel, with a P wave following the third beat and preceding the fifth beat. This is an

example of sinus rhythm with AV dissociation and anterior concordance due to ventricular tachycardia. Coded 6, 27, and 50.

14. This patient has what appears to be a posterolateral infarct. However, the delta waves throughout make this an example of sinus rhythm with Wolff-Parkinson-White syndrome. Coded 4 and 47.

15. This patient has a right bundle branch block. The ST segment is distorted by late occurrence of the P waves, and there are inferior and lateral Q waves caused by infarctions in the inferior and lateral leads. This is a nodule or junctional rhythm with retrograde activation of the atrium, right bundle branch block, and infarcts on the lateral and inferior walls. Coded 21, 55, 77, 78, and 94.

Exercise IV

ANSWER SHEET
Exercise IV

Patient 1   ——   ——   ——   ——   ——   ——   ——   ——

Patient 2   ——   ——   ——   ——   ——   ——   ——   ——

Patient 3   ——   ——   ——   ——   ——   ——   ——   ——

Patient 4   ——   ——   ——   ——   ——   ——   ——   ——

Patient 5   ——   ——   ——   ——   ——   ——   ——   ——

Patient 6   ——   ——   ——   ——   ——   ——   ——   ——

Patient 7   ——   ——   ——   ——   ——   ——   ——   ——

Patient 8   ——   ——   ——   ——   ——   ——   ——   ——

Patient 9   ——   ——   ——   ——   ——   ——   ——   ——

Patient 10   ——   ——   ——   ——   ——   ——   ——   ——

Patient 11   ——   ——   ——   ——   ——   ——   ——   ——

Patient 12   ——   ——   ——   ——   ——   ——   ——   ——

Patient 13   ——   ——   ——   ——   ——   ——   ——   ——

Patient 14   ——   ——   ——   ——   ——   ——   ——   ——

Patient 15   ——   ——   ——   ——   ——   ——   ——   ——

Electrocardiographic Diagnostic Coding Sheet

General Features
1. Normal ECG
2. Normal ECG, variant
3. Misplaced leads
4. Electrical alternans

Sinus Rhythms
5. Normal sinus
6. Sinus tachycardia
7. Sinus bradycardia
8. Sinus arrhythmia
9. Sinus pause or arrest

Atrial Rhythms
10. Premature atrial contractions (PAC)
11. Aberrant PAC
12. Ectopic atrial rhythm
13. Atrial tachycardia with AV block
14. Atrial fibrillation
15. Atrial flutter
16. Multifocal atrial tachycardia
17. Dual atrial rhythms

AV Junctional Rhythms
18. Premature junctional beats (PJB)
19. Aberrant PJB
20. Junctional beat or rhythm
21. AV junctional rhythm with retrograde atrial activation
22. Supraventricular tachycardia

Ventricular Rhythms
23. Premature ventricular contractions (PVC), unifocal
24. PVC, multifocal
25. PVC, couplets/triplets
26. PVC, R-on-T phenomenon

27. Ventricular tachycardia
28. Idioventricular rhythm
29. Ventricular fibrillation
30. Ventricular escape beat or rhythm
31. Ventricular fusion beat or rhythm
32. Ventricular capture beat during VT
33. Torsades de pointes

Pacemaker Rhythms
34. Fixed rate
35. Demand
36. Atrial pacing
37. Ventricular pacing
38. Dual chamber pacing
39. Failure to sense
40. Failure to capture

AV Conduction Abnormalities
41. 1° AV block
42. Wenckebach (Mobitz I) AV block
43. 2° AV block (Mobitz II)
44. Fixed 2° AV block, 2:1, 4:1, etc.
45. Complete heart block
46. Variable AV block
47. Preexcitation (WPW)

AV - VA Interactions
48. Fusion beat
49. Echo beat
50. AV dissociation
51. Isorhythmic AV dissociation

Intraventricular Conduction Abnormalities
52. Left axis

53. Right axis
54. Incomplete RBBB
55. Complete RBBB
56. Incomplete LBBB
57. Complete LBBB
58. Anterior hemiblock
59. Posterior hemiblock
60. Nonspecific IVCD
61. Arrhythmia related aberrancy
62. Intermittent IVCD/BBB

Chamber Enlargement
63. Left atrial enlargement
64. Right atrial enlargement
65. Bi-atrial enlargement
66. LVH - voltage
67. LVH - voltage plus repolarization changes
68. RVH
69. Biventricular hypertrophy

Myocardial Infarction

Recent/Acute
70. Anteroseptal
71. Anterior
72. Lateral
73. Inferior
74. Posterior

Old/Uncertain Age
75. Anteroseptal
76. Anterior
77. Lateral
78. Inferior
79. Posterior

Repolarization Changes
80. Possible LV aneurysm
81. Non-Q wave infarction

82. Early repolarization
83. Persistent juvenile T wave
84. ST-T wave changes of acute injury
85. ST-T wave changes of acute ischemia
86. ST-T wave changes of hypertrophy or altered intraventricular conduction (secondary repolarization changes)
87. ST-T wave changes of pericarditis
88. ST changes due to digitalis effect
89. Nonspecific ST-T wave changes
90. Postectopic T wave changes
91. Peaked T waves
92. Prolonged QT interval
93. Prominent U waves

Clinical Problems
94. Coronary artery disease
95. Congenital heart disease
96. Mitral valve disease
97. Hyperkalemia
98. Hypokalemia
99. Hypercalcemia
100. Hypocalcemia
101. Digitalis toxicity
102. CNS event
103. Motion artifact
104. Dextrocardia
105. Cardiac tamponade
106. Cardiac transplant
107. Chronic lung disease

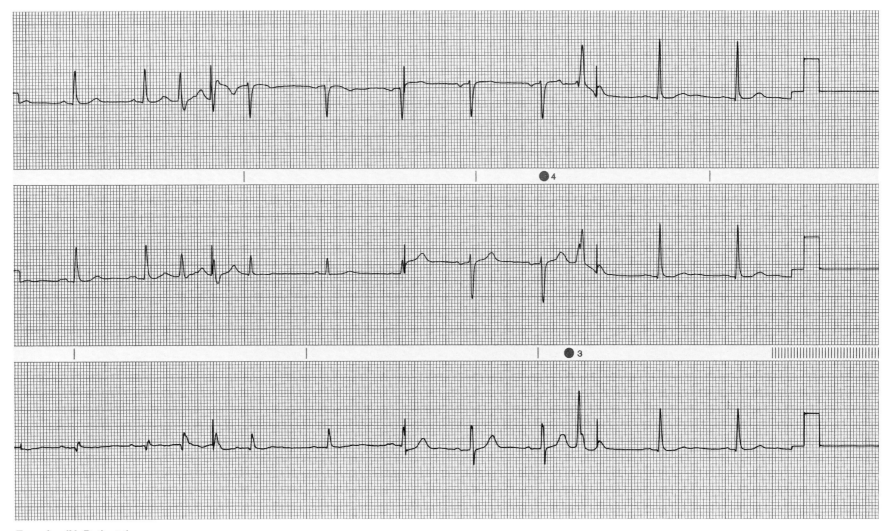

Exercise IV, Patient 1

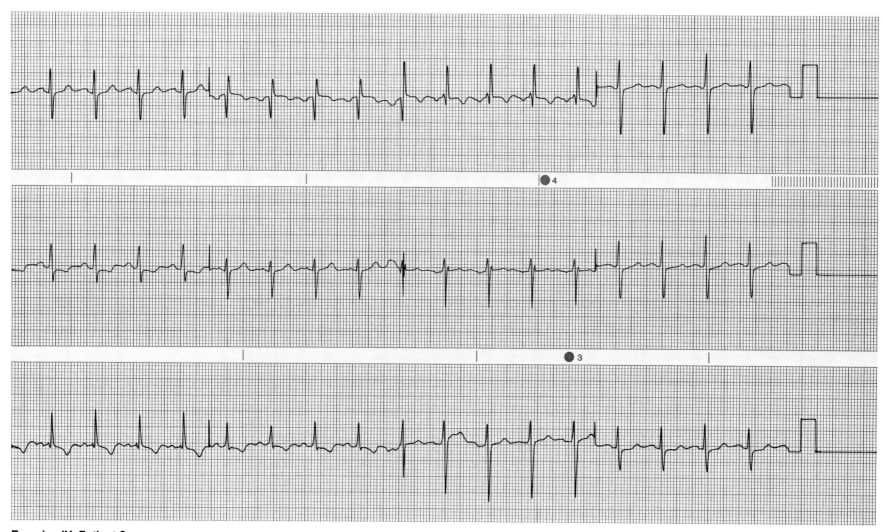

Exercise IV, Patient 2

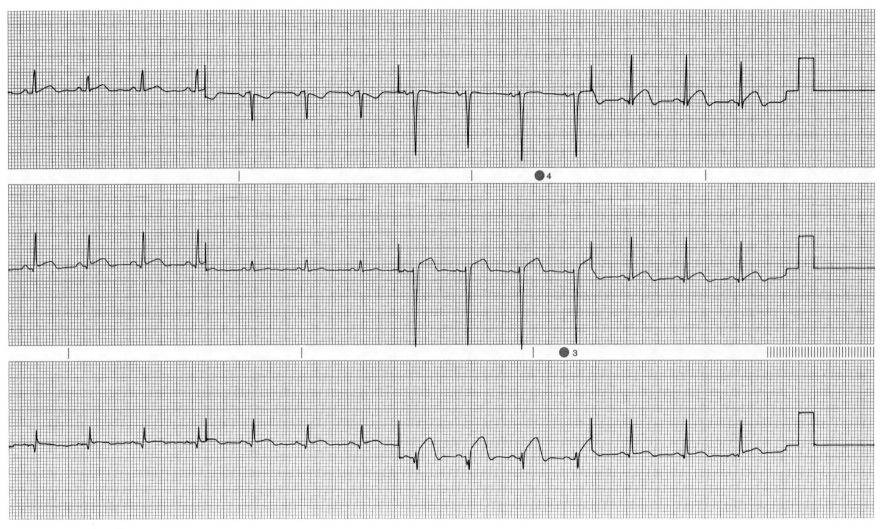

Exercise IV, Patient 3

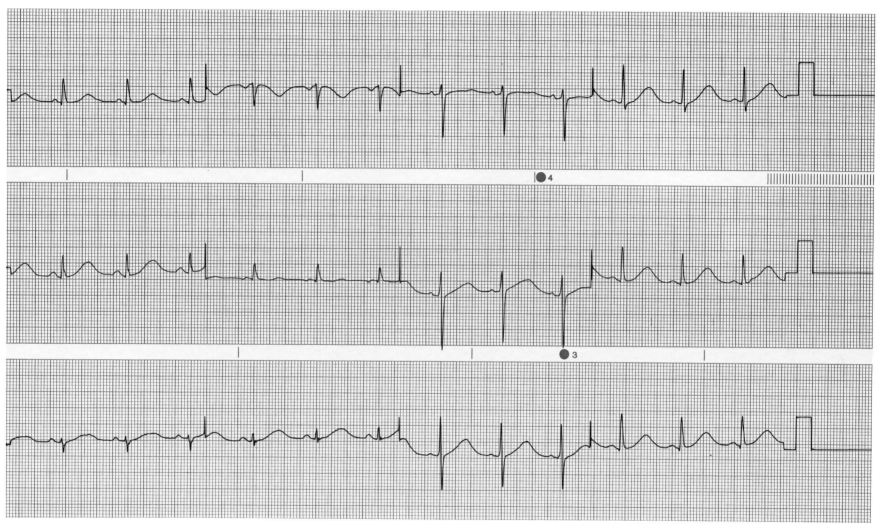

Exercise IV, Patient 4

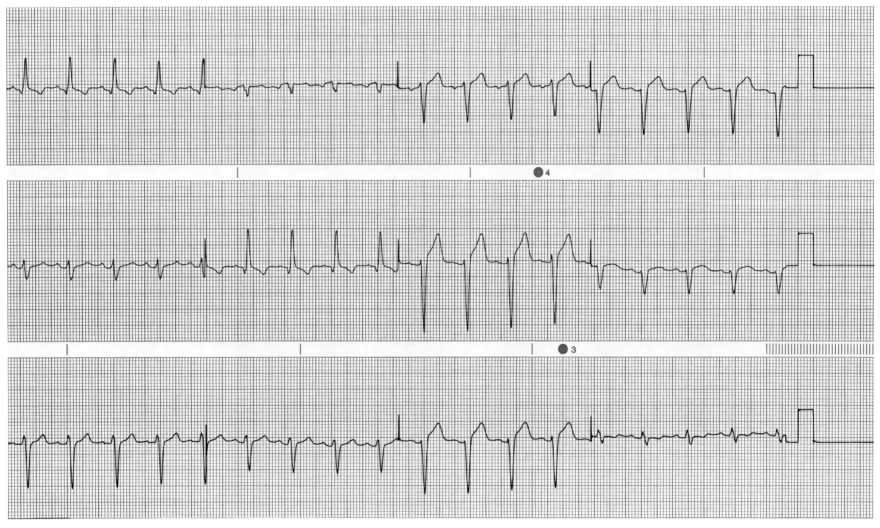

Exercise IV, Patient 5

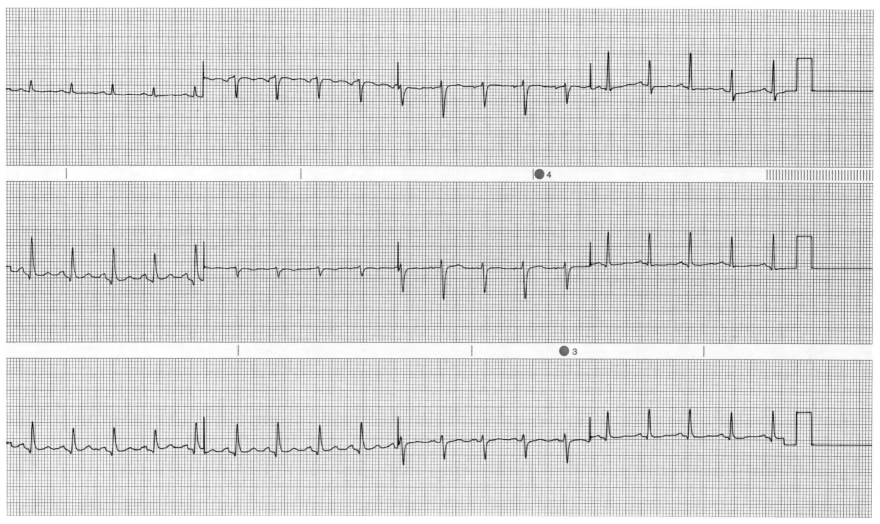

Exercise IV, Patient 6

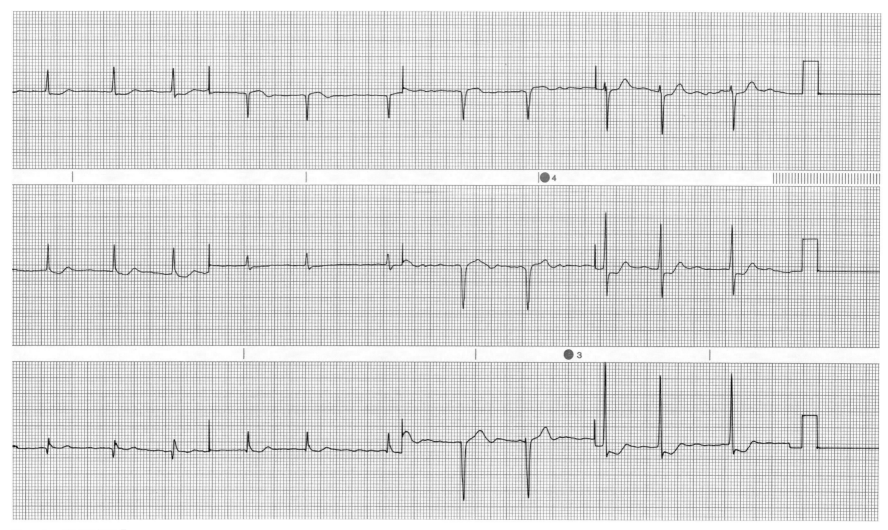

Exercise IV, Patient 7

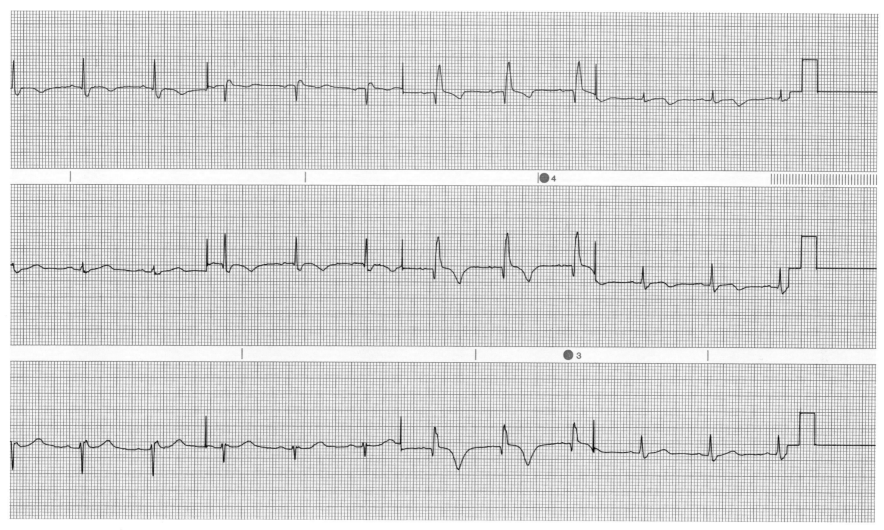

Exercise IV, Patient 8

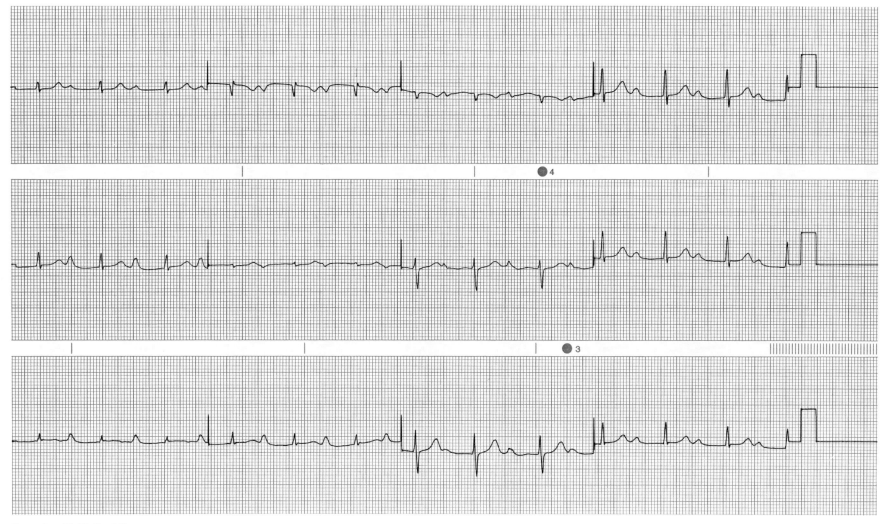

Exercise IV, Patient 9

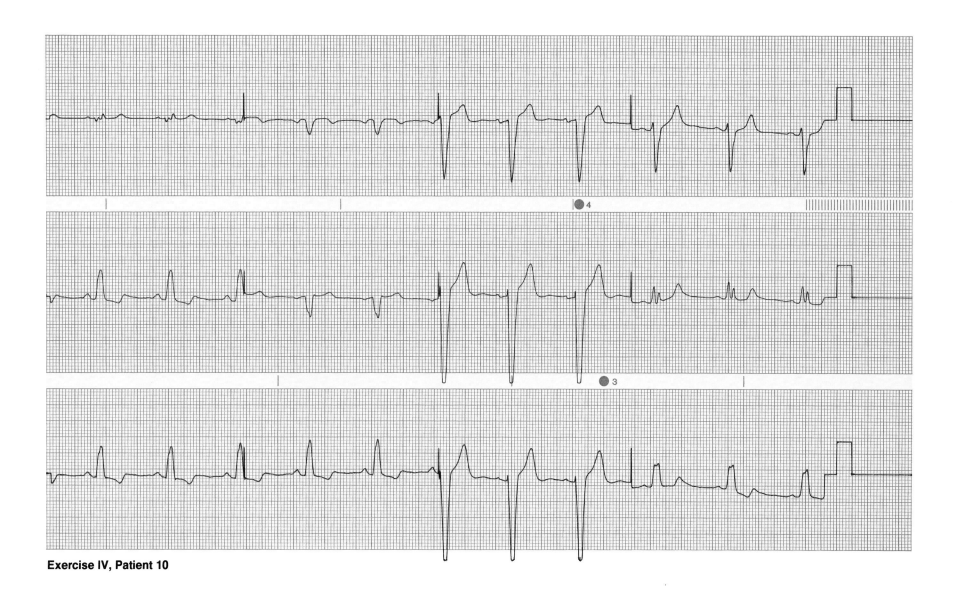

Exercise IV, Patient 10

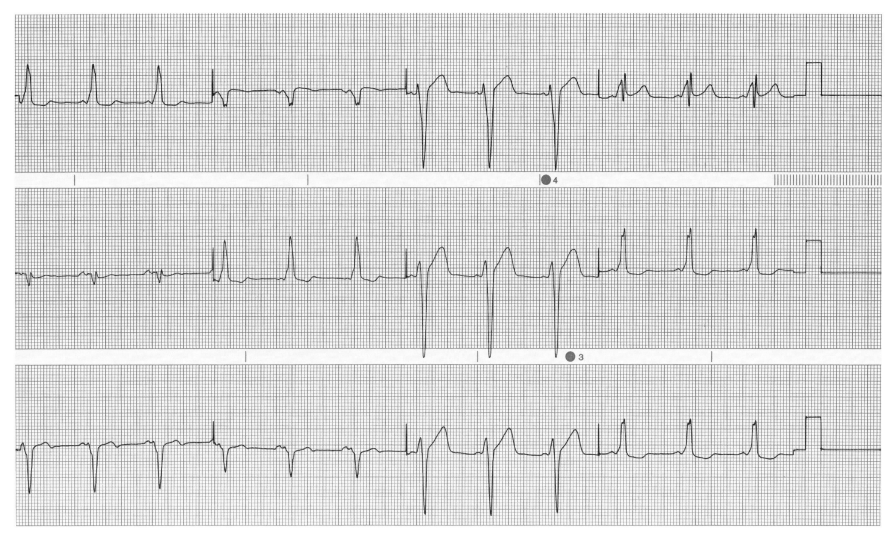

Exercise IV, Patient 11

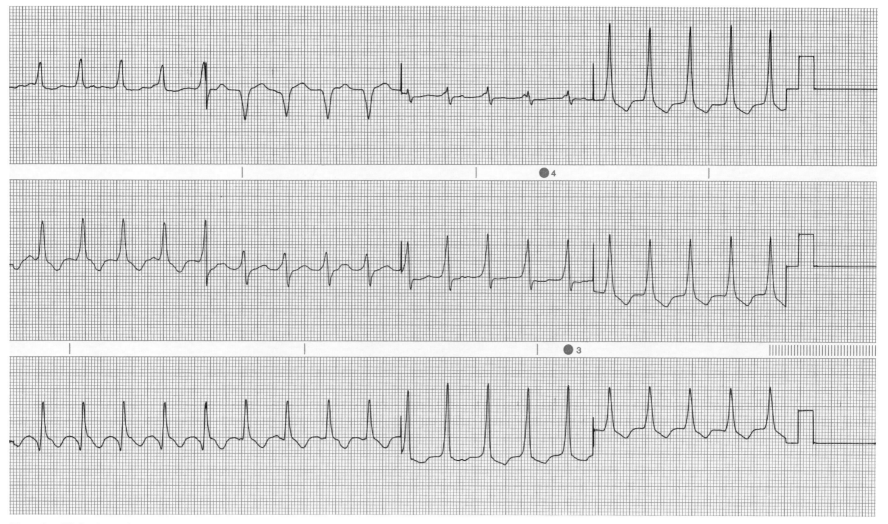

Exercise IV, Patient 12

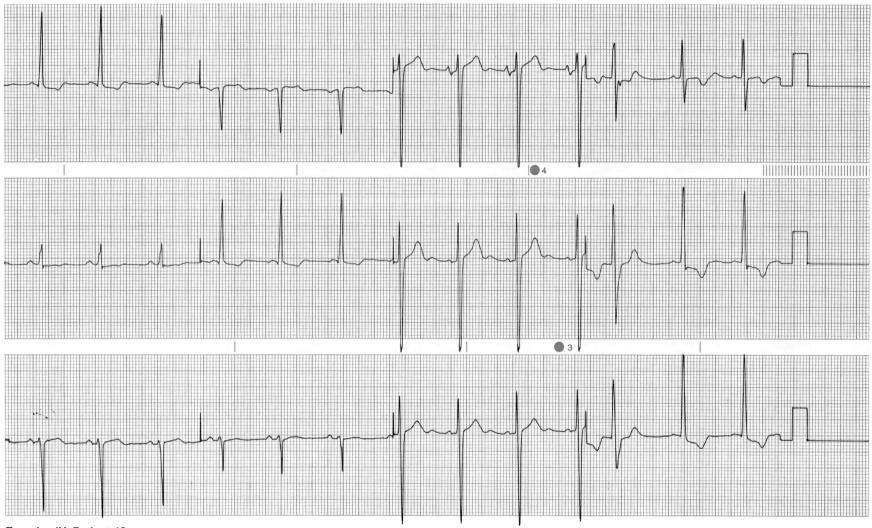

Exercise IV, Patient 13

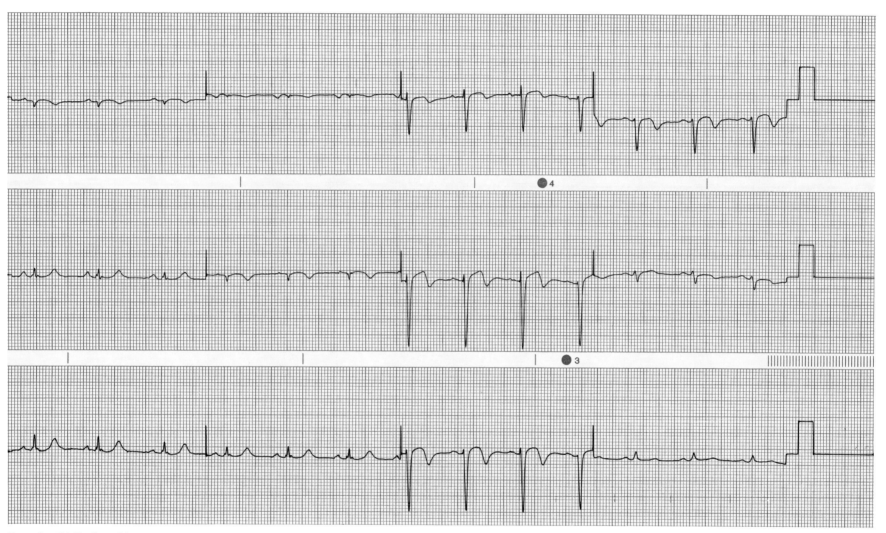

Exercise IV, Patient 14

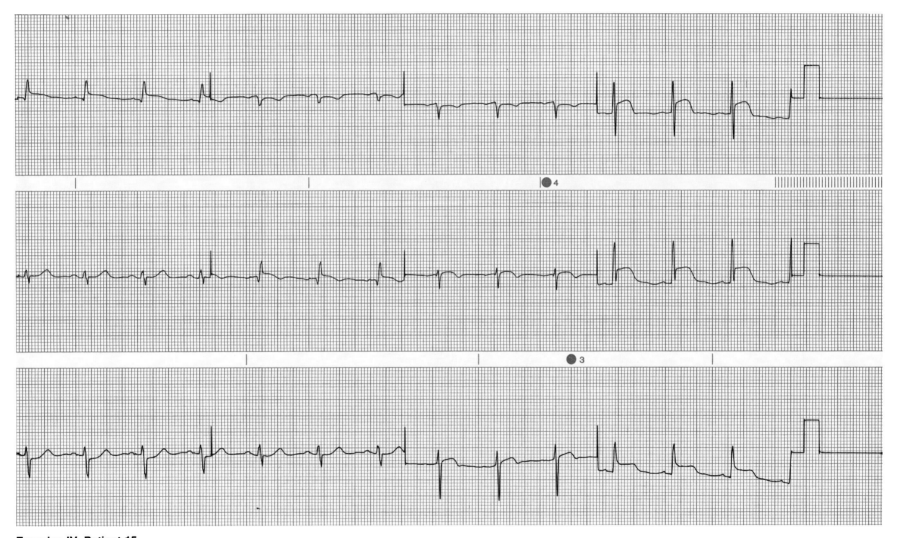

Exercise IV, Patient 15

1. This electrocardiogram shows a sinus rhythm with aberrantly conducted premature atrial contractions and possibly left atrial enlargement. The premature atrial contractions (PACs) with aberrancy are most clearly seen in the third panel. This right bundle branch block configuration tends to be the case with aberrancy. There are paired PACs at the end and beginning of panels 1 and 2, respectively. A prolonged P wave with notching in lead II suggests left atrial enlargement. Coded 5, 11, and 63.

2. This patient has a sinus rhythm, an incomplete right bundle branch block, and right ventricular hypertrophy, established by the RSR′ pattern with R′ > S in lead V₁. In addition, the R:S ratio is <1 in leads V₅ and V₆, supporting a diagnosis of right ventricular hypertrophy. There is right axis deviation, as evidenced by equalization of the positive and negative forces in lead I. Coded 6, 53, 54, and 68.

3. This patient has normal sinus rhythm and acute anterior (and probably acute inferior) infarctions. The ST segment elevation is obvious in the mid precordial leads. Also there is ST segment elevation in leads II and aV_F with terminal T wave abnormalities. This type of pattern is not infrequently seen with occlusion of wide-ranging, left anterior descending coronary arteries. Coded 5, 71, 73, 84, and 94.

4. This electrocardiogram shows broadening of the QT interval. This is a nonspecific finding in this case since it is the only abnormality on the electrocardiogram. Coded 5 and 92.

5. This is an example of poor R wave progression caused by myocardial infarction. There actually is R wave regression with the force of the initial positive vector being less in lead V₃ than in lead V₂. There is a broad Q wave in lead aV_L, which is consistent with an anterolateral infarct. The electrocardiogram also shows anterior hemiblock with marked left axis deviation and typical changes in the aV_L lead. Coded 6, 58, 76, 77, and 94.

6. This electrocardiogram shows sinus tachycardia, electrical alternans, and nonspecific ST-T wave changes or nonspecific repolarization changes. This combination suggests cardiac tamponade. Coded 4, 6, 89, and 105.

7. This patient has atrial fibrillation, an old anteroseptal infarction, and repolarization changes from digitalis. There is scooping ST segment depression in leads II and V₆ with shortening of the QT interval consistent with digitalis effect. There are Q waves in leads V₁ and V₂, and a qrS pattern in lead V₃, which supports the diagnosis of anteroseptal infarct. Coded 14, 75, 88, and 94.

8. This is a right bundle branch block with an old anteroseptal infarction. There are also a sinus rhythm and nonspecific repolarization changes. The right bundle branch block is diagnosed by the broad R wave in lead V₁ and broad terminal S in lead V₆. The infarct is supported by the Q waves in leads V₁ through V₃ in the face of right bundle branch block. There is leftward axis but not enough to call an anterior hemiblock. Coded 5, 52, 55, 75, 89, and 94.

9. This is an abnormal electrocardiogram caused by a first-degree AV block. The patient has a sinus rhythm and a very prolonged PR interval. Coded 5 and 41.

10. This patient has a left bundle branch block and a sinus rhythm. There are broad QRS complexes >120 milliseconds and no Q waves in leads V₆ or I. Coded 5 and 57.

11. This electrocardiogram suggests left bundle branch block but, in fact, is preexcitation, as evidenced by the delta waves, which are especially noted laterally. The underlying rhythm is sinus. Coded 5 and 47.

12. This electrocardiogram has a wide QRS complex in leads V₆ and I without Q waves. It is a regular rhythm and might suggest sinus rhythm with left bundle branch block, except that there is AV dissociation with P waves following the second beat in panel 3 and just before the fourth beat in panel 3. This indicates ventricular tachycardia. Coded 6, 27, and 50.

13. This electrocardiogram has prominent lateral forces. There are tiny Q waves in leads I and V₆, and there is a fairly typical lateral strain pattern consistent with left ventricular hypertrophy. The first beat in the fourth panel has a distorted P wave and a slightly different depolarization pattern, indicating an aberrant premature atrial contraction. Coded 5, 11, and 67.

14. This electrocardiogram shows an anterolateral infarction of uncertain age. There is persistent ST segment elevation in the precordial leads and terminal symmetry of the T waves. This may be seen in the chronic phase of an infarction but is more suggestive of a recent event. There are precordial R wave regression and Q waves in leads I and aV_L, which by themselves are not diagnostic but if taken with leads V₄ and V₅ suggest anterolateral infarct. Coded 5, 71, 72, 84, and 94.

15. This is a typical acute anterior and lateral infarct. There is ST segment elevation in leads I, aV_L, and V₃ to V₆. Coded 5, 71, 72, 84, and 94.

Exercise V

ANSWER SHEET
Exercise V

Patient 1   —— —— —— —— —— —— —— ——

Patient 2   —— —— —— —— —— —— —— ——

Patient 3   —— —— —— —— —— —— —— ——

Patient 4   —— —— —— —— —— —— —— ——

Patient 5   —— —— —— —— —— —— —— ——

Patient 6   —— —— —— —— —— —— —— ——

Patient 7   —— —— —— —— —— —— —— ——

Patient 8   —— —— —— —— —— —— —— ——

Patient 9   —— —— —— —— —— —— —— ——

Patient 10   —— —— —— —— —— —— —— ——

Patient 11   —— —— —— —— —— —— —— ——

Patient 12   —— —— —— —— —— —— —— ——

Patient 13   —— —— —— —— —— —— —— ——

Patient 14   —— —— —— —— —— —— —— ——

Patient 15   —— —— —— —— —— —— —— ——

Electrocardiographic Diagnostic Coding Sheet

General Features
1. Normal ECG
2. Normal ECG, variant
3. Misplaced leads
4. Electrical alternans

Sinus Rhythms
5. Normal sinus
6. Sinus tachycardia
7. Sinus bradycardia
8. Sinus arrhythmia
9. Sinus pause or arrest

Atrial Rhythms
10. Premature atrial contractions (PAC)
11. Aberrant PAC
12. Ectopic atrial rhythm
13. Atrial tachycardia with AV block
14. Atrial fibrillation
15. Atrial flutter
16. Multifocal atrial tachycardia
17. Dual atrial rhythms

AV Junctional Rhythms
18. Premature junctional beats (PJB)
19. Aberrant PJB
20. Junctional beat or rhythm
21. AV junctional rhythm with retrograde atrial activation
22. Supraventricular tachycardia

Ventricular Rhythms
23. Premature ventricular contractions (PVC), unifocal
24. PVC, multifocal
25. PVC, couplets/triplets
26. PVC, R-on-T phenomenon
27. Ventricular tachycardia
28. Idioventricular rhythm
29. Ventricular fibrillation
30. Ventricular escape beat or rhythm
31. Ventricular fusion beat or rhythm
32. Ventricular capture beat during VT
33. Torsades de pointes

Pacemaker Rhythms
34. Fixed rate
35. Demand
36. Atrial pacing
37. Ventricular pacing
38. Dual chamber pacing
39. Failure to sense
40. Failure to capture

AV Conduction Abnormalities
41. 1° AV block
42. Wenckebach (Mobitz I) AV block
43. 2° AV block (Mobitz II)
44. Fixed 2° AV block, 2:1, 4:1, etc.
45. Complete heart block
46. Variable AV block
47. Preexcitation (WPW)

AV - VA Interactions
48. Fusion beat
49. Echo beat
50. AV dissociation
51. Isorhythmic AV dissociation

Intraventricular Conduction Abnormalities
52. Left axis
53. Right axis
54. Incomplete RBBB
55. Complete RBBB
56. Incomplete LBBB
57. Complete LBBB
58. Anterior hemiblock
59. Posterior hemiblock
60. Nonspecific IVCD
61. Arrhythmia related aberrancy
62. Intermittent IVCD/BBB

Chamber Enlargement
63. Left atrial enlargement
64. Right atrial enlargement
65. Bi-atrial enlargement
66. LVH - voltage
67. LVH - voltage plus repolarization changes
68. RVH
69. Biventricular hypertrophy

Myocardial Infarction

Recent/Acute
70. Anteroseptal
71. Anterior
72. Lateral
73. Inferior
74. Posterior

Old/Uncertain Age
75. Anteroseptal
76. Anterior
77. Lateral
78. Inferior
79. Posterior

Repolarization Changes
80. Possible LV aneurysm
81. Non-Q wave infarction
82. Early repolarization
83. Persistent juvenile T wave
84. ST-T wave changes of acute injury
85. ST-T wave changes of acute ischemia
86. ST-T wave changes of hypertrophy or altered intraventricular conduction (secondary repolarization changes)
87. ST-T wave changes of pericarditis
88. ST changes due to digitalis effect
89. Nonspecific ST-T wave changes
90. Postectopic T wave changes
91. Peaked T waves
92. Prolonged QT interval
93. Prominent U waves

Clinical Problems
94. Coronary artery disease
95. Congenital heart disease
96. Mitral valve disease
97. Hyperkalemia
98. Hypokalemia
99. Hypercalcemia
100. Hypocalcemia
101. Digitalis toxicity
102. CNS event
103. Motion artifact
104. Dextrocardia
105. Cardiac tamponade
106. Cardiac transplant
107. Chronic lung disease

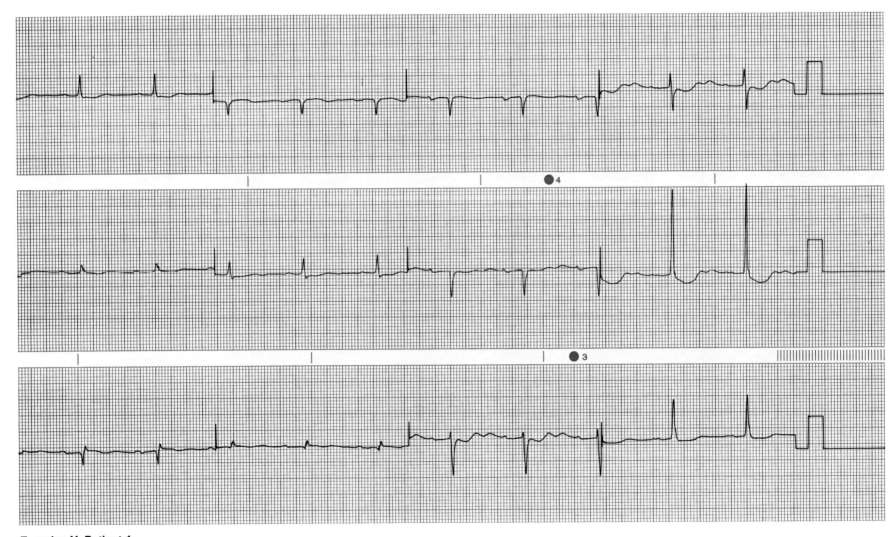

Exercise V, Patient 1

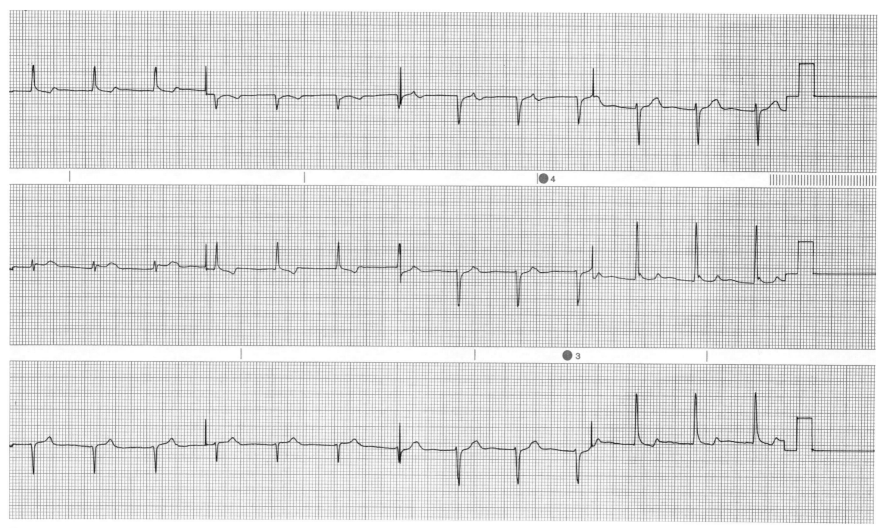

Exercise V, Patient 2

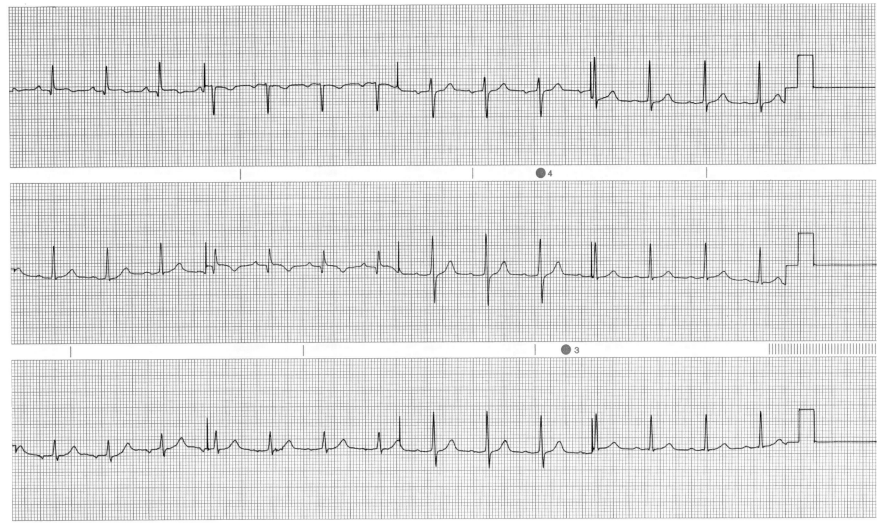

Exercise V, Patient 3

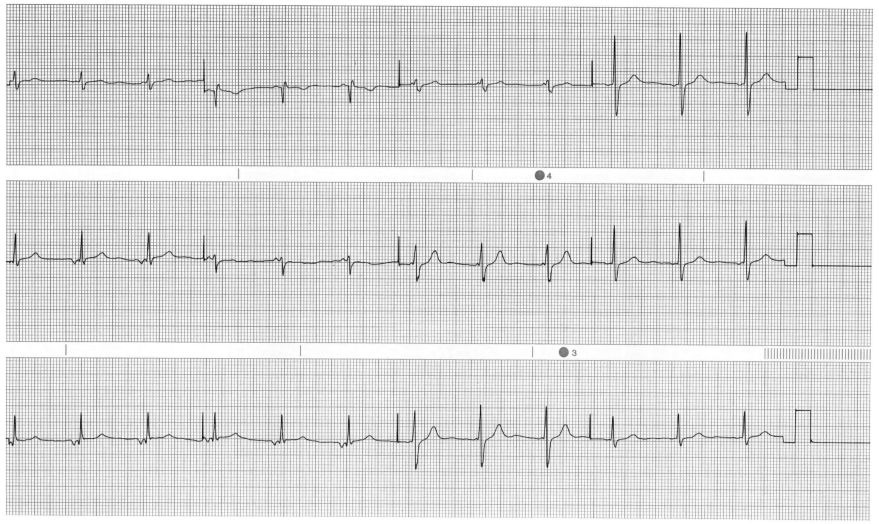

Exercise V, Patient 4

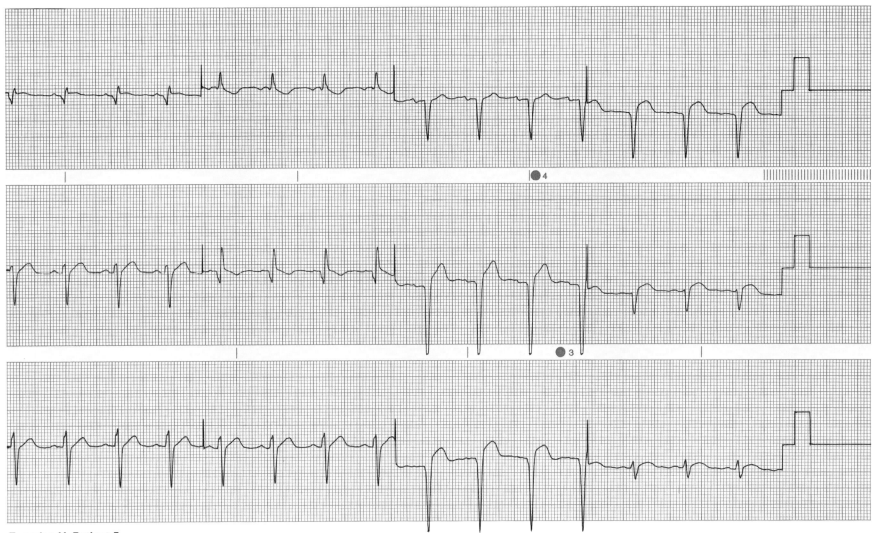

Exercise V, Patient 5

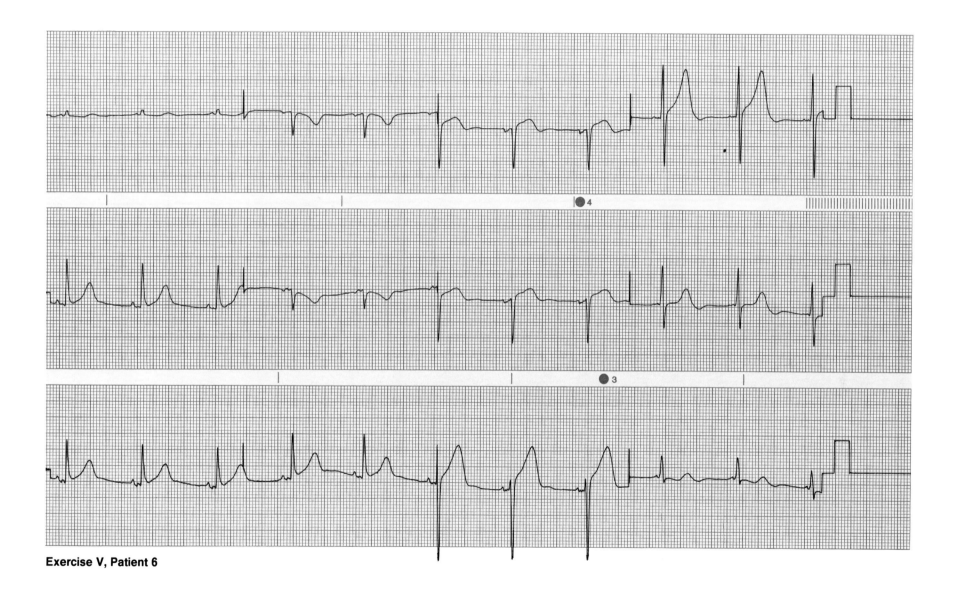

Exercise V, Patient 6

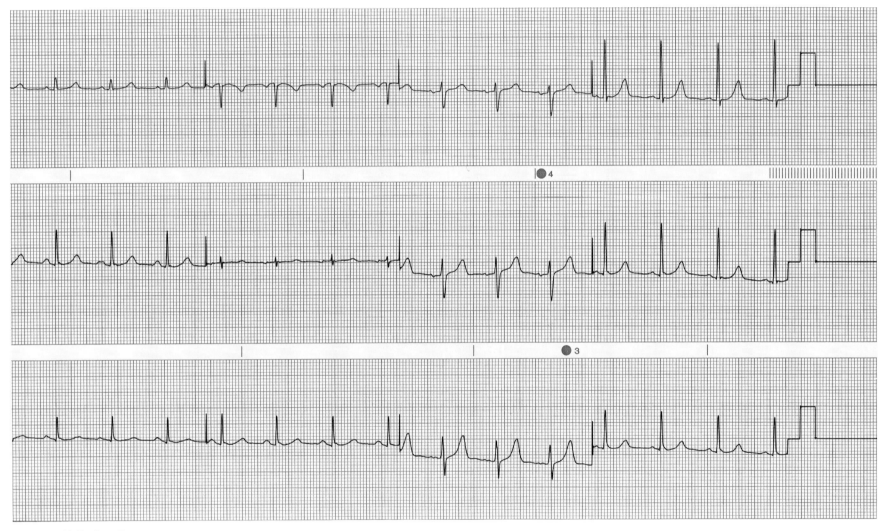

Exercise V, Patient 7

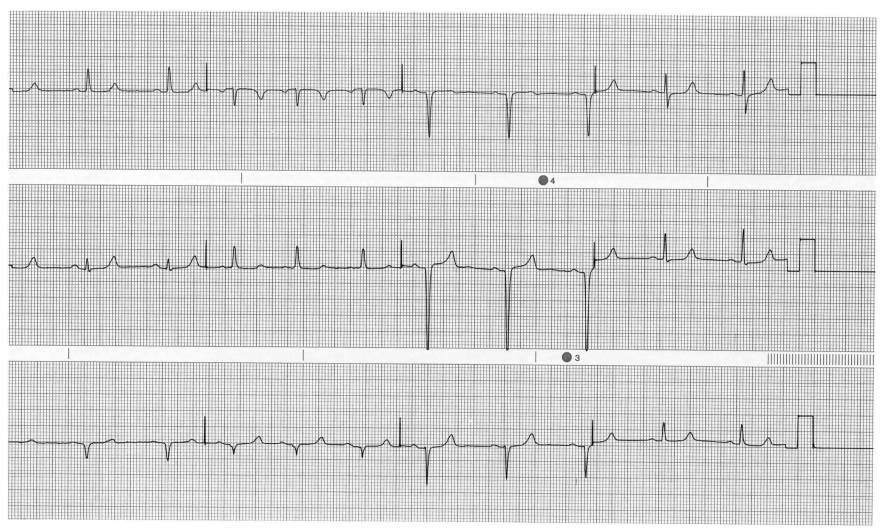

Exercise V, Patient 8

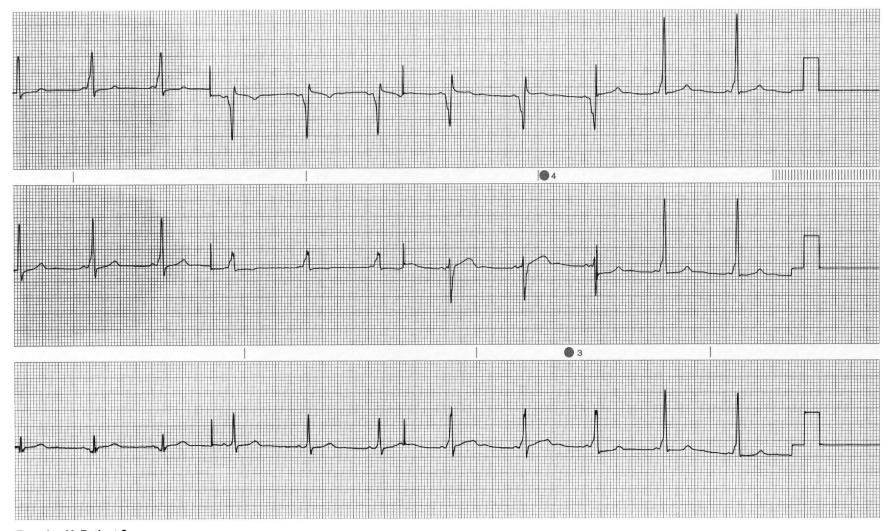

Exercise V, Patient 9

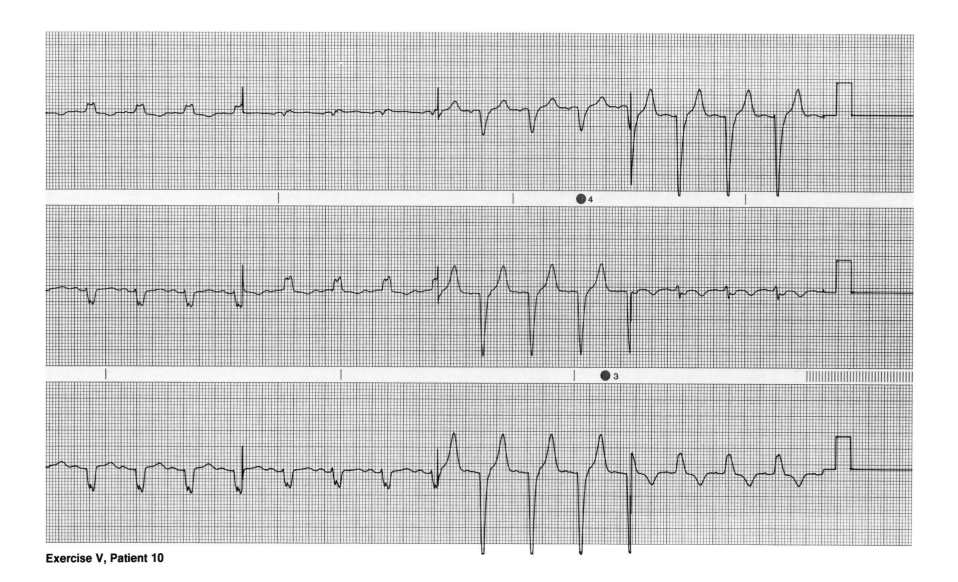

Exercise V, Patient 10

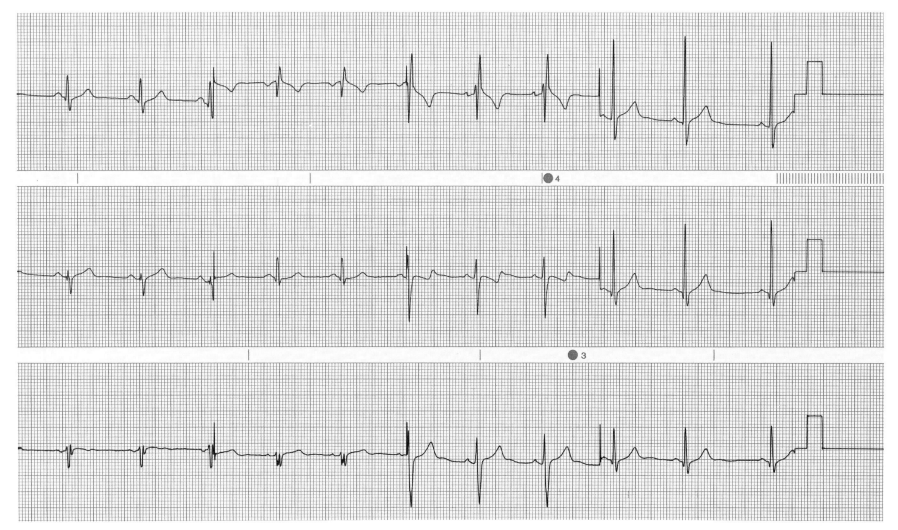

Exercise V, Patient 11

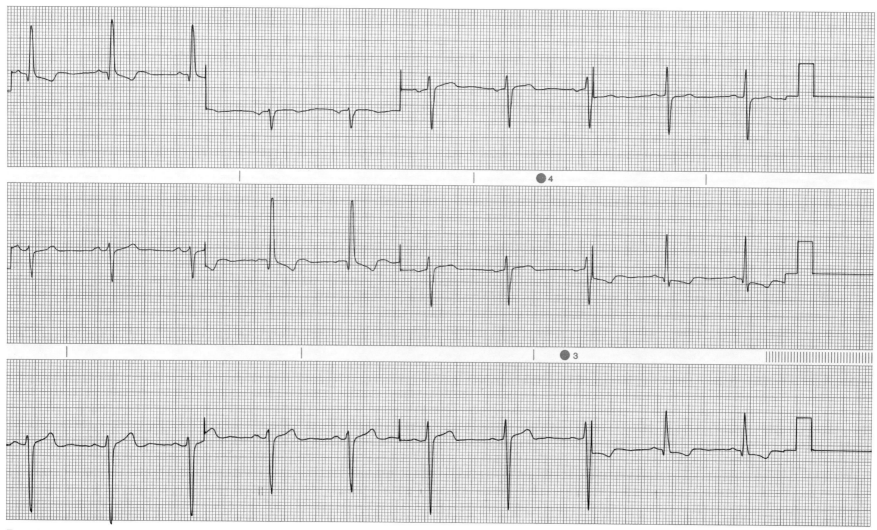

Exercise V, Patient 12

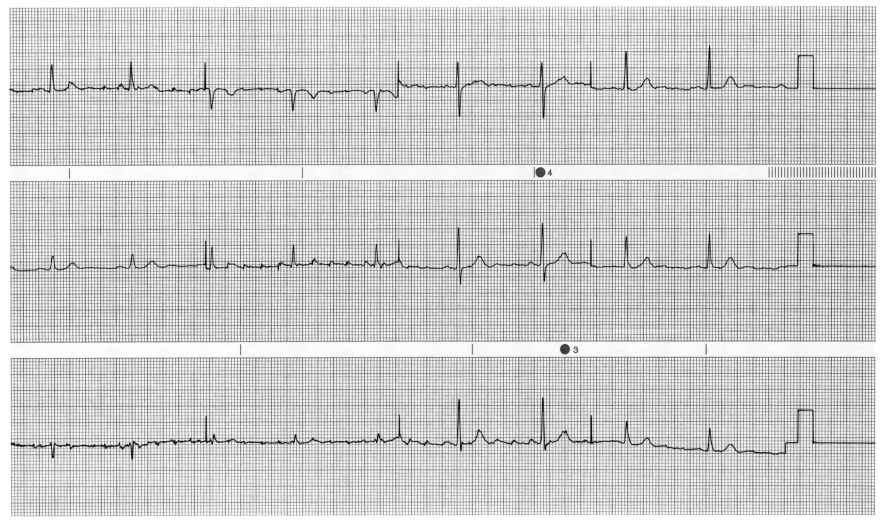

Exercise V, Patient 13

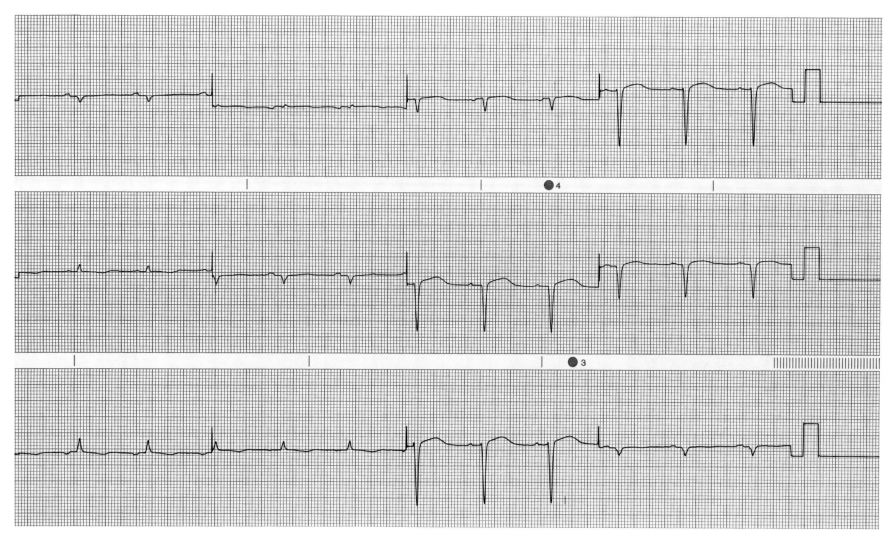

Exercise V, Patient 14

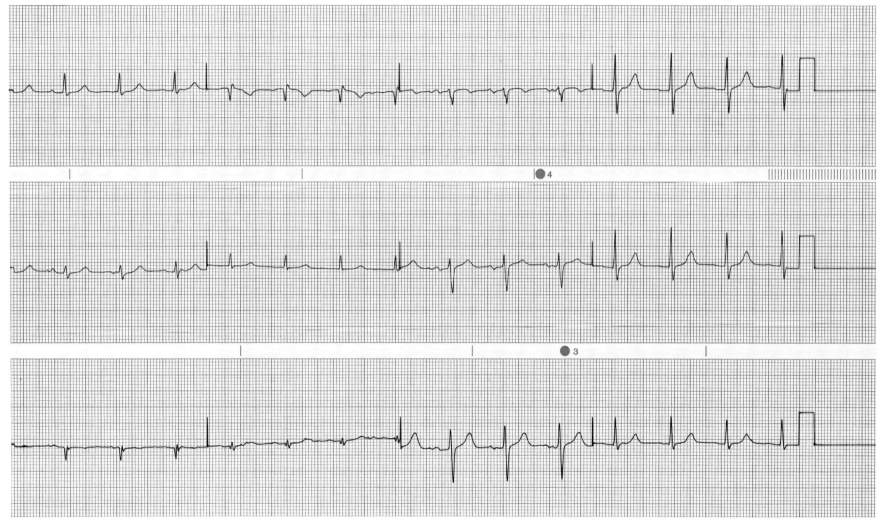

Exercise V, Patient 15

1. This electrocardiogram shows a sinus rhythm with a first-degree AV block and hypokalemia. The ST segments are depressed. There is prominence of the U waves, especially in leads V_3 and V_4. Coded 5, 41, 93, and 98.

2. This patient has a junctional rhythm with retrograde activation of the atria. There are also nonspecific lateral repolarization abnormalities. Coded 21 and 89.

3. This is a high lateral myocardial infarction with Q waves and T wave changes in lead aV_L. The age is uncertain. This infarct developed silently after hip surgery. Coded 5, 77, and 94.

4. This electrocardiogram is normal except for an abnormal P wave axis, suggesting low atrial or junctional rhythm. Coded 12.

5. This electrocardiogram shows a sinus rhythm. It has extensive Q waves of an anterolateral infarction and a marked left axis with a QRS complex < 120 milliseconds, consistent with an anterior hemiblock. There are ST segment elevations associated with well-developed Q waves. If the infarct was a remote event, this would raise the possibility of a ventricular aneurysm. Coded 5, 58, 76, 77, 80, and 94.

6. This patient has a sinus rhythm and an acute anterior infarction. ST segments are elevated in the right and mid precordium, and the T waves have become wide with symmetry (hyperacute T waves). This is early in the acute phase of the infarct. Coded 5, 70, 84, and 94.

7. This electrocardiogram is normal. Coded 1 (and possibly 5).

8. This electrocardiogram shows relative prolongation of the QT interval with a symmetric quality of the T waves. There also are inferiorly directed Q waves in lead III and especially in lead aV_F. This is a sinus rhythm with an inferior infarct and possibly hypocalcemia. Coded 5, 78, 92, 94, and 100.

9. This electrocardiogram shows preexcitation. Delta waves and short PR intervals are obvious. Coded 5 and 47.

10. This patient has a sinus rhythm, left axis, and left bundle branch block. The QRS complex is broad, there are secondary repolarization changes in the lateral leads, and no Q waves in leads I, V_6, or aV_L. Coded 5, 52, 57, and 86.

11. This patient has congenital heart disease with an atrial septal defect. There is an RSR′ pattern in lead V_1, which is not broad, so a diagnosis of incomplete right bundle branch block is made. R′ > S establishes right ventricular hypertrophy. Coded 5, 52, 54, 68, and 95.

12. This patient has ventricular hypertrophy. The QRS complex is broad and > 120 milliseconds, but there are Q waves in leads I and V_6, giving a diagnosis of intraventricular delay rather than complete left bundle branch block. Voltage in lead aV_L is tall; there are secondary T wave changes plus left axis. Because of the width of the QRS complex, anterior hemiblock should not be diagnosed. Coded 7, 52, 60, and 67.

13. This patient has a sinus rhythm and a tremor. The R wave in lead V_1 is prominent. This plus an upright T wave raises the possibility of an old posterior infarct. Clinically, Parkinson's disease was present. Coded 5 and 103 (and possibly 79 and 94).

14. This patient has a sinus rhythm with extensive Q waves in leads V_2 through V_6, I, and aV_L caused by myocardial infarct. Coded 5, 76, 77, and 94.

15. This is the same patient after cardiac transplantation. R forces are back to normal. There is a sinus rhythm as well as an accessory atrial rhythm dissociated from the rest of the cardiac activity. These P waves can most clearly be seen in the third panel (preceding the first P wave and following the third P wave) and in the first panel (following the second P wave and distorting the first P wave). This is a second atrial rhythm of cardiac transplantation and should be identified. Coded 17 and 106.

Exercise VI

ANSWER SHEET
Exercise VI

Patient 1   —— —— —— —— —— —— —— ——

Patient 2   —— —— —— —— —— —— —— ——

Patient 3   —— —— —— —— —— —— —— ——

Patient 4   —— —— —— —— —— —— —— ——

Patient 5   —— —— —— —— —— —— —— ——

Patient 6   —— —— —— —— —— —— —— ——

Patient 7   —— —— —— —— —— —— —— ——

Patient 8   —— —— —— —— —— —— —— ——

Patient 9   —— —— —— —— —— —— —— ——

Patient 10   —— —— —— —— —— —— —— ——

Patient 11   —— —— —— —— —— —— —— ——

Patient 12   —— —— —— —— —— —— —— ——

Patient 13   —— —— —— —— —— —— —— ——

Patient 14   —— —— —— —— —— —— —— ——

Patient 15   —— —— —— —— —— —— —— ——

Electrocardiographic Diagnostic Coding Sheet

General Features
1. Normal ECG
2. Normal ECG, variant
3. Misplaced leads
4. Electrical alternans

Sinus Rhythms
5. Normal sinus
6. Sinus tachycardia
7. Sinus bradycardia
8. Sinus arrhythmia
9. Sinus pause or arrest

Atrial Rhythms
10. Premature atrial contractions (PAC)
11. Aberrant PAC
12. Ectopic atrial rhythm
13. Atrial tachycardia with AV block
14. Atrial fibrillation
15. Atrial flutter
16. Multifocal atrial tachycardia
17. Dual atrial rhythms

AV Junctional Rhythms
18. Premature junctional beats (PJB)
19. Aberrant PJB
20. Junctional beat or rhythm
21. AV junctional rhythm with retrograde atrial activation
22. Supraventricular tachycardia

Ventricular Rhythms
23. Premature ventricular contractions (PVC), unifocal
24. PVC, multifocal
25. PVC, couplets/triplets
26. PVC, R-on-T phenomenon
27. Ventricular tachycardia
28. Idioventricular rhythm
29. Ventricular fibrillation
30. Ventricular escape beat or rhythm
31. Ventricular fusion beat or rhythm
32. Ventricular capture beat during VT
33. Torsades de pointes

Pacemaker Rhythms
34. Fixed rate
35. Demand
36. Atrial pacing
37. Ventricular pacing
38. Dual chamber pacing
39. Failure to sense
40. Failure to capture

AV Conduction Abnormalities
41. 1° AV block
42. Wenckebach (Mobitz I) AV block
43. 2° AV block (Mobitz II)
44. Fixed 2° AV block, 2:1, 4:1, etc.
45. Complete heart block
46. Variable AV block
47. Preexcitation (WPW)

AV - VA Interactions
48. Fusion beat
49. Echo beat
50. AV dissociation
51. Isorhythmic AV dissociation

Intraventricular Conduction Abnormalities
52. Left axis
53. Right axis
54. Incomplete RBBB
55. Complete RBBB
56. Incomplete LBBB
57. Complete LBBB
58. Anterior hemiblock
59. Posterior hemiblock
60. Nonspecific IVCD
61. Arrhythmia related aberrancy
62. Intermittent IVCD/BBB

Chamber Enlargement
63. Left atrial enlargement
64. Right atrial enlargement
65. Bi-atrial enlargement
66. LVH - voltage
67. LVH - voltage plus repolarization changes
68. RVH
69. Biventricular hypertrophy

Myocardial Infarction
Recent/Acute
70. Anteroseptal
71. Anterior
72. Lateral
73. Inferior
74. Posterior

Old/Uncertain Age
75. Anteroseptal
76. Anterior
77. Lateral
78. Inferior
79. Posterior

Repolarization Changes
80. Possible LV aneurysm
81. Non-Q wave infarction
82. Early repolarization
83. Persistent juvenile T wave
84. ST-T wave changes of acute injury
85. ST-T wave changes of acute ischemia
86. ST-T wave changes of hypertrophy or altered intraventricular conduction (secondary repolarization changes)
87. ST-T wave changes of pericarditis
88. ST changes due to digitalis effect
89. Nonspecific ST-T wave changes
90. Postectopic T wave changes
91. Peaked T waves
92. Prolonged QT interval
93. Prominent U waves

Clinical Problems
94. Coronary artery disease
95. Congenital heart disease
96. Mitral valve disease
97. Hyperkalemia
98. Hypokalemia
99. Hypercalcemia
100. Hypocalcemia
101. Digitalis toxicity
102. CNS event
103. Motion artifact
104. Dextrocardia
105. Cardiac tamponade
106. Cardiac transplant
107. Chronic lung disease

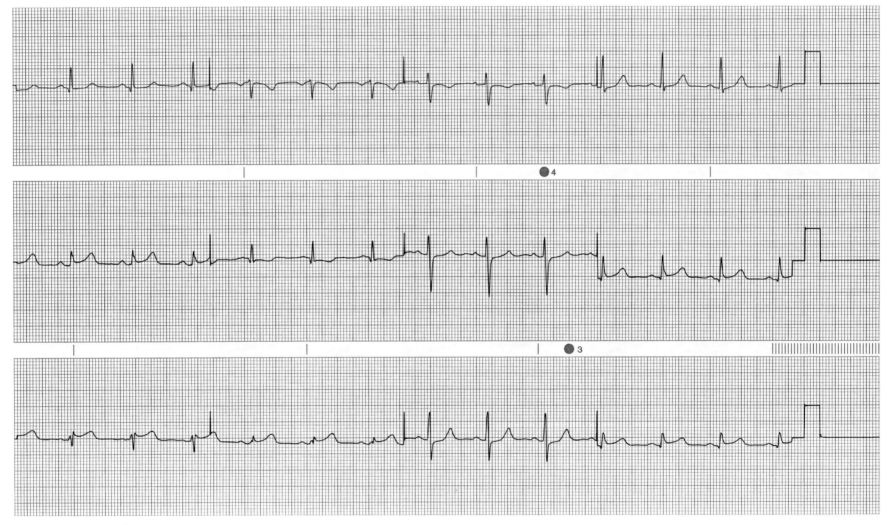

Exercise VI, Patient 1

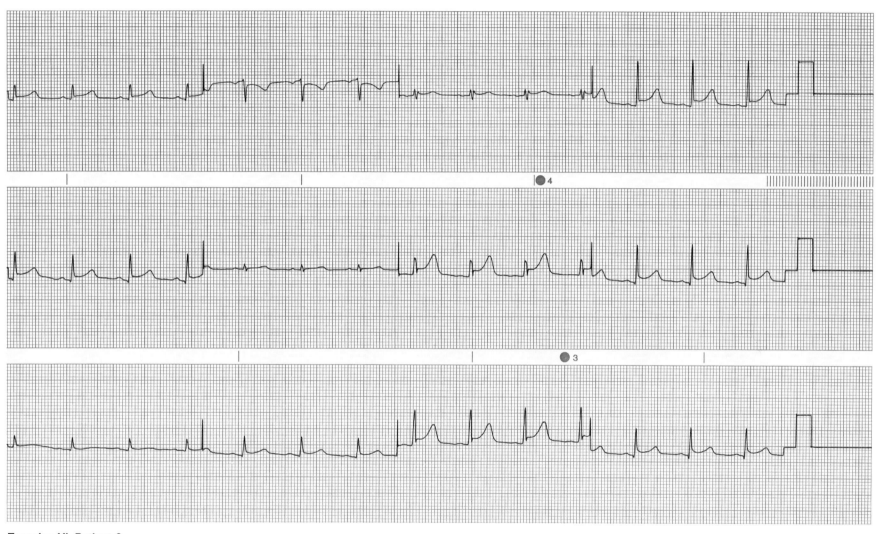

Exercise VI, Patient 2

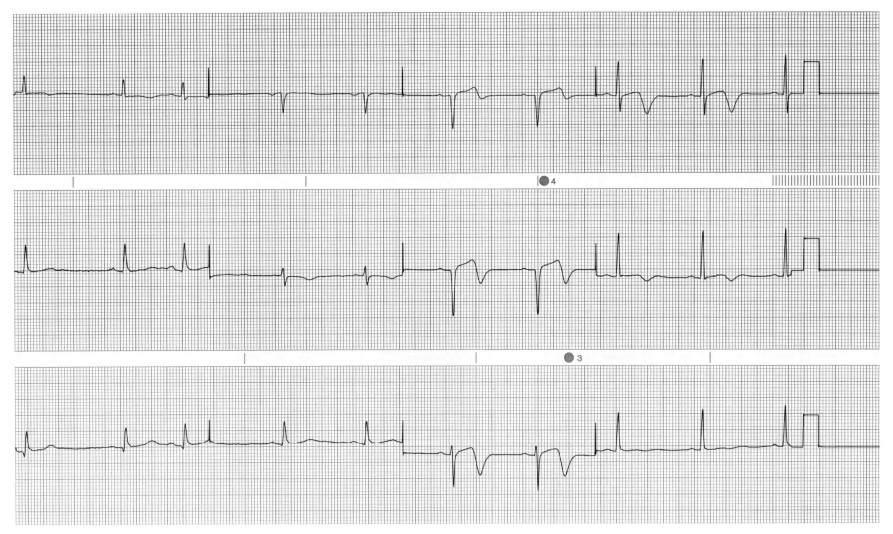

Exercise VI, Patient 3

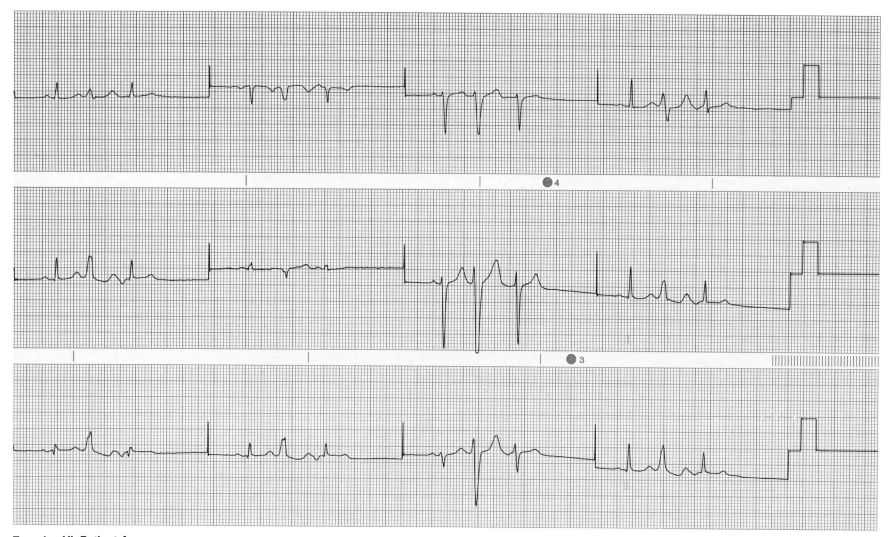

Exercise VI, Patient 4

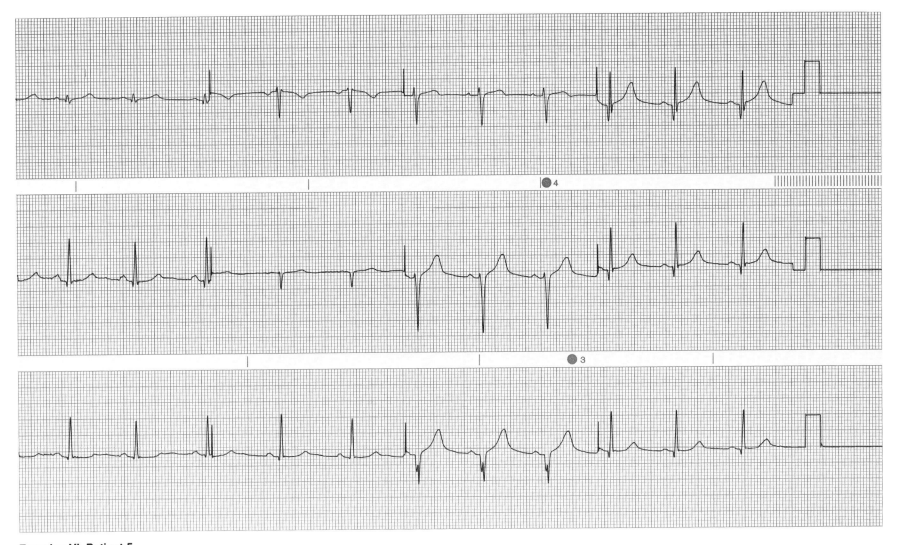

Exercise VI, Patient 5

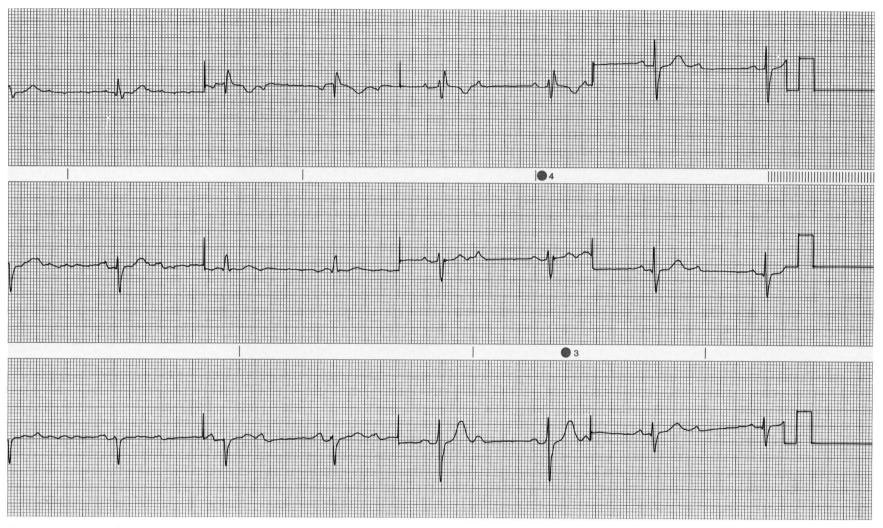

Exercise VI, Patient 6

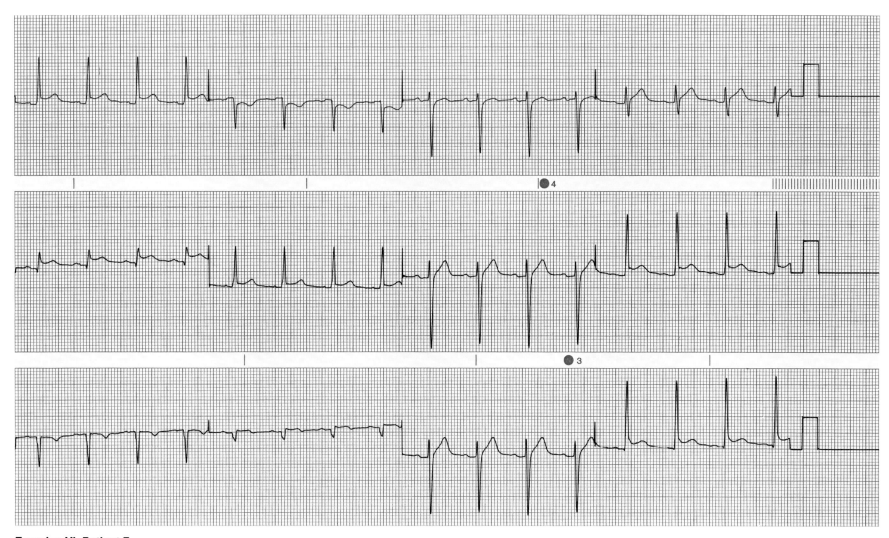

Exercise VI, Patient 7

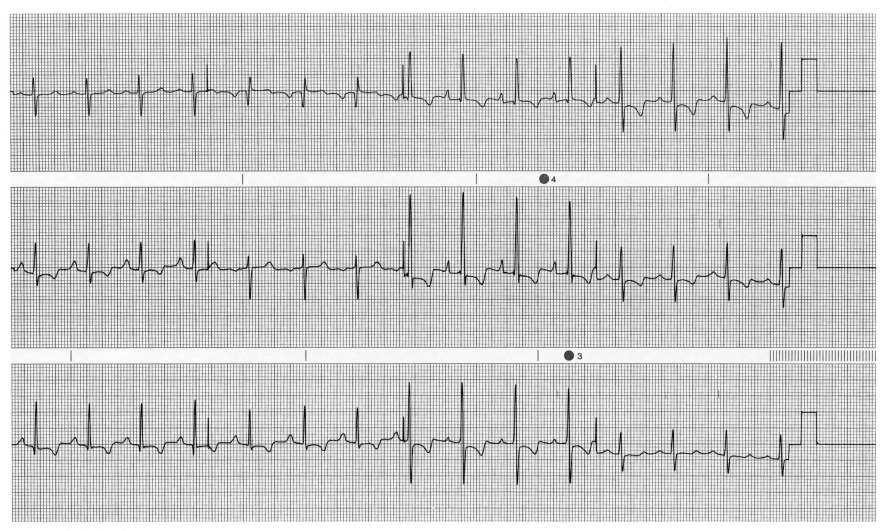

Exercise VI, Patient 8

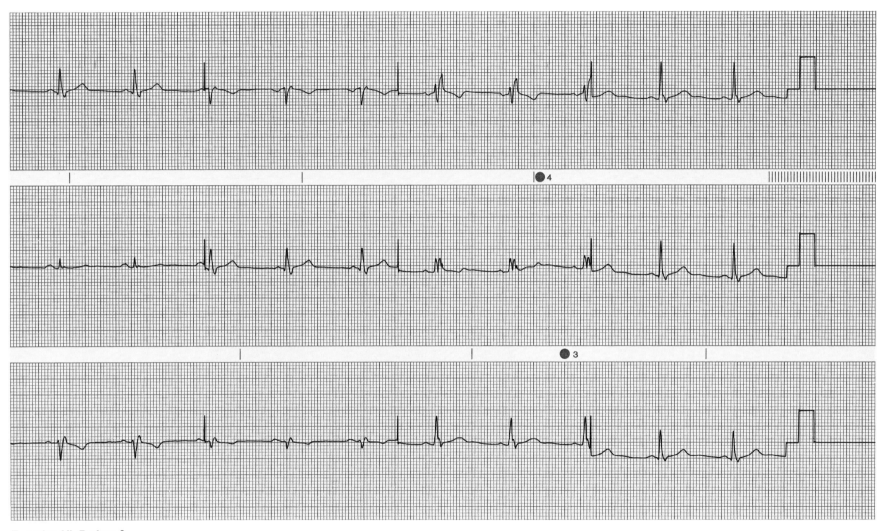

Exercise VI, Patient 9

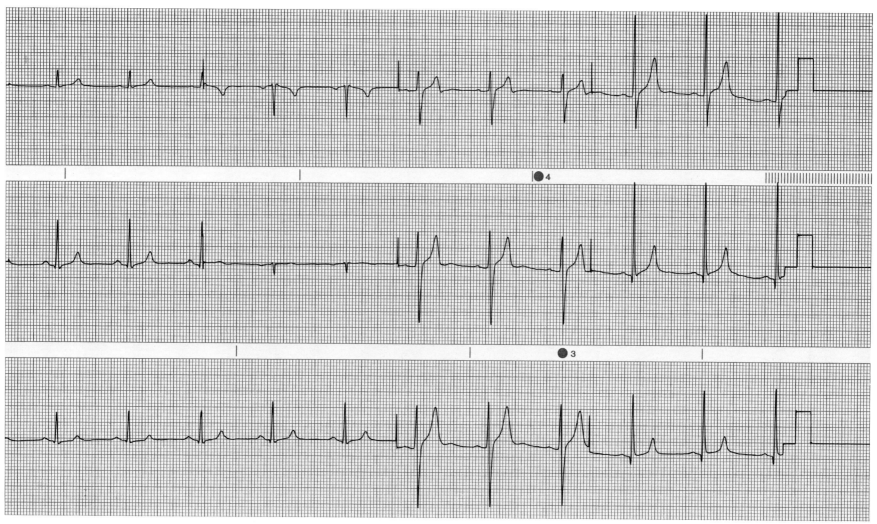

Exercise VI, Patient 10

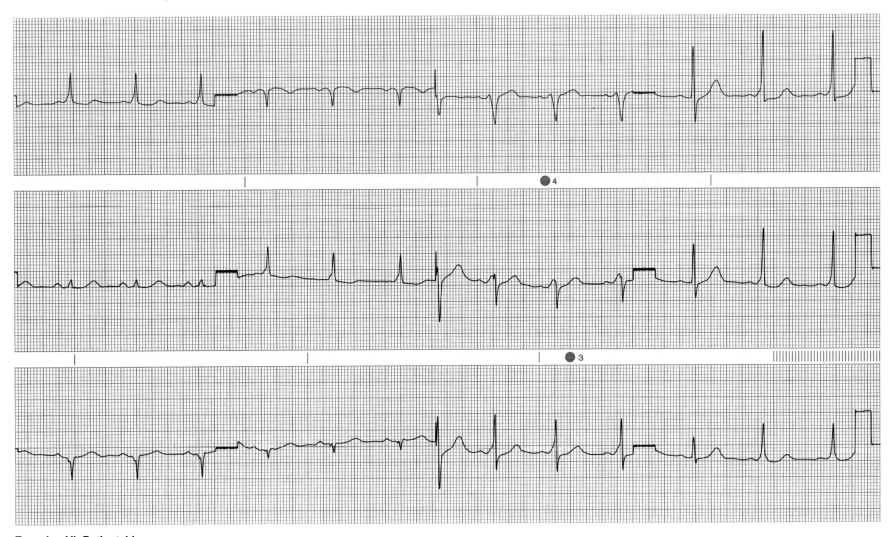

Exercise VI, Patient 11

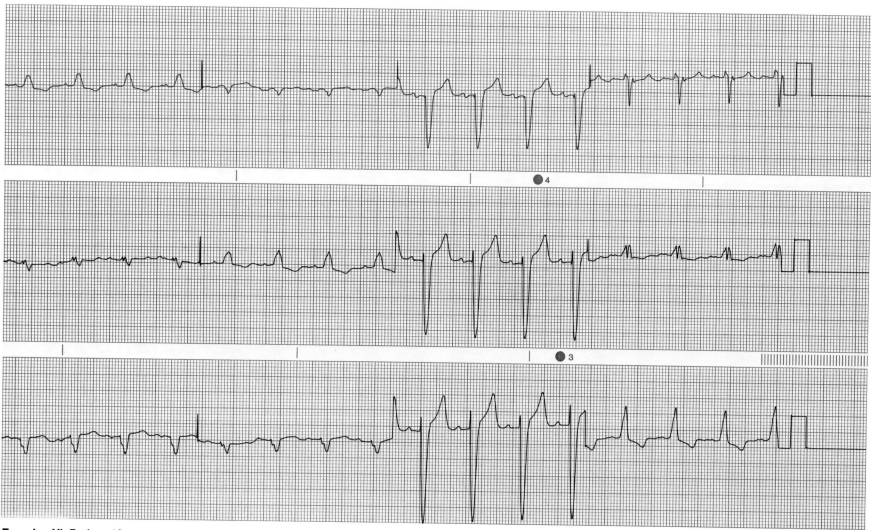

Exercise VI, Patient 12

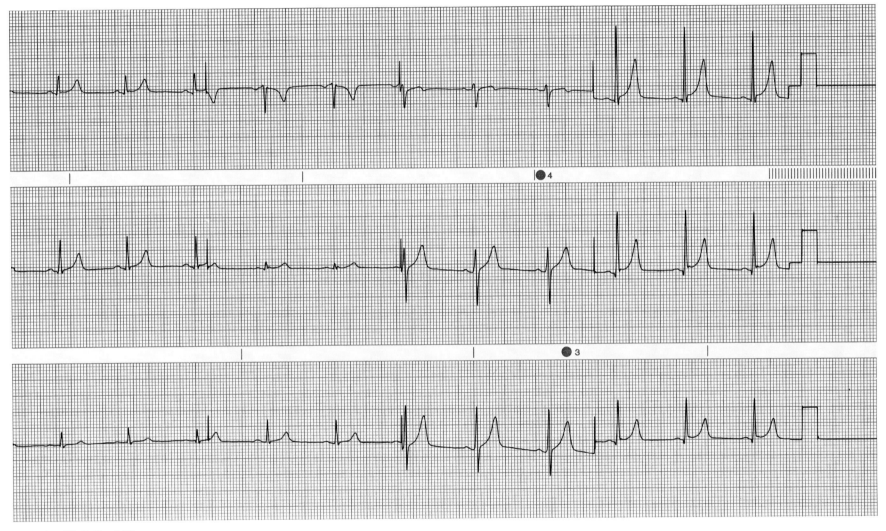

Exercise VI, Patient 13

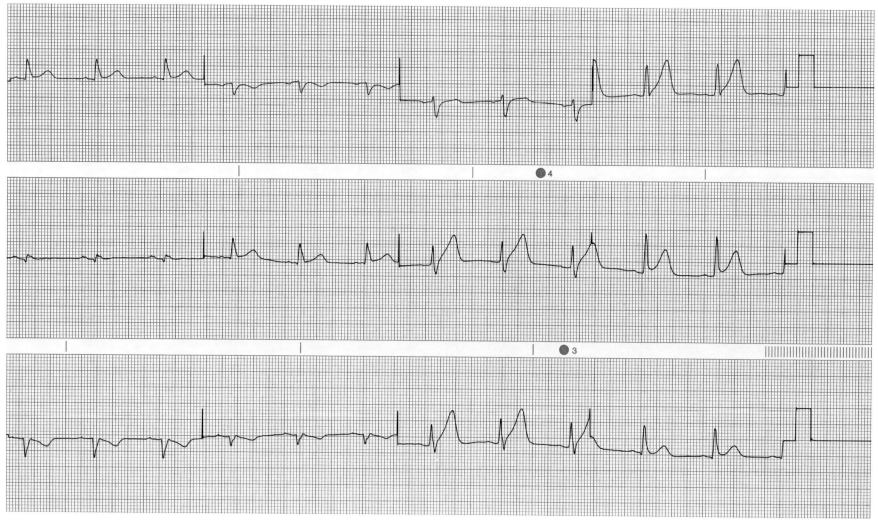

Exercise VI, Patient 14

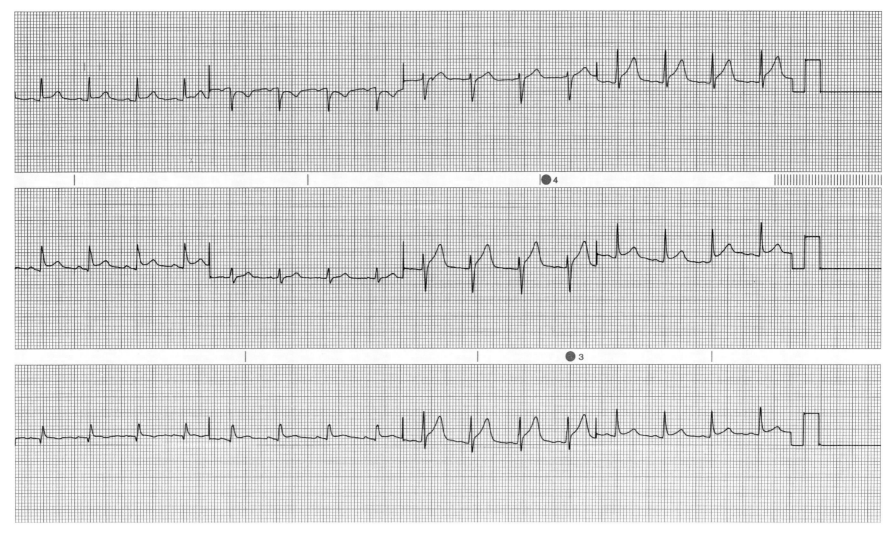

Exercise VI, Patient 15

1. This was a young diabetic who smoked and ultimately died of coronary disease. This shows her first infarction, which was an acute inferior event. There is ST segment elevation in leads II, III, aV_F, and V_6 and reciprocal depression in lead aV_L. Coded 5, 73, 84, and 94.

2. This electrocardiogram shows a normal sinus rhythm. An RSR′ pattern in lead V_1 suggests incomplete right bundle branch block, and generalized ST segment elevation is consistent with pericarditis. In pericarditis, ST segments commonly are depressed in lead aV_R, may be depressed or isoelectric in lead V_1, and occasionally are isoelectric in leads aV_L and III. Coded 5, 54, and 87. Since R is > than S in V_1, it is not impossible that a posterior infarct is also present in this patient. Coded 79 and 94.

3. This patient has terminal symmetry of the T waves in the mid precordial leads, consistent with a non–Q wave infarction. In addition, the third beat is a premature atrial contraction. There are nonspecific lateral ST-T wave changes. Coded 7, 10, 81, 89, and 94.

4. This is an example of group beating. The sequence is made up of sinus beats followed by premature ventricular contractions, then echo beats initiated by inverted P waves, and all followed by a sinus pause before the whole sequence repeats itself. Coded 5, 9, 23, and 49.

5. This is an old anterior infarction showing R wave regression into a Q wave in lead V_3. Coded 5, 76, and 94.

6. This patient has a sinus rhythm with a 2:1 AV block, a complete right bundle branch block, left anterior hemiblock, and motion artifact evident in the extremity leads. The right bundle branch block is establish by the late R′ and T wave changes in lead V_1 and the broad terminal S in lead V_6. Marked left axis and a characteristic small Q wave in aV_L establish the diagnosis of anterior hemiblock. The 2:1 AV block is best seen in the third panel. Coded 5, 43, 44, 55, 58, 86, and 103.

7. This patient has a clear inferior infarct. The Q wave is broad and deep in lead aV_F and is supported by Q waves in lead II and III. In addition, there is ST segment elevation in most leads except V_1, aV_R and III. This is consistent with acute pericarditis. Coded 5, 78, 87, and 94.

8. This electrocardiogram shows rSR′ with prominent R′ in lead V_1, consistent with right ventricular hypertrophy. Right axis deviation supports this. There are changes also of right atrial enlargement with a positive prominence of the P waves in leads II, V_1, and V_2. Coded 5, 53, 64, 68, and 86.

9. This is a sinus rhythm with right bundle branch block. Coded 5, 55, and 86.

10. This electrocardiogram shows narrow symmetric prominence of the T waves, especially in the lateral precordial leads, and raises the possibility of hyperkalemia. In fact, this patient with renal insufficiency had elevated potassium before dialysis. Coded 5, 91, and 97.

11. This patient has intermittent Wolff-Parkinson-White syndrome. Most beats are conducted with preexcitated fusion, except for a premature contraction initiating the third panel and the first beat in the forth panel, which is normally conducted. Coded 5 and 47.

12. This is a left bundle branch block. The QRS complex is broad and >120 milliseconds in the standard limb leads. There are secondary T wave changes evident, especially in leads I, aV_L, and V_6. There is an absence of Q waves in leads I and V_6. Coded 5, 57, and 86.

13. This patient has ST segment elevation and prominence of the T waves. These are asymmetric, however. The best diagnosis here is early repolarization, a normal variant. Coded 2, 5, and 82.

14. This electrocardiogram also shows some ST segment elevation. The T waves also are prominent. They are somewhat symmetric and are broad. This is most consistent with acute anterior infarct. In addition, there are inferiorly directed Q waves of an old inferior infarct. Coded 5, 71, 78, 84, and 94.

15. This electrocardiogram also shows ST segment elevation but is diffuse in quality and consistent with acute pericarditis. Coded 6 and 87.

Exercise VII

ANSWER SHEET
Exercise VII

Patient 1   ___ ___ ___ ___ ___ ___ ___ ___

Patient 2   ___ ___ ___ ___ ___ ___ ___ ___

Patient 3   ___ ___ ___ ___ ___ ___ ___ ___

Patient 4   ___ ___ ___ ___ ___ ___ ___ ___

Patient 5   ___ ___ ___ ___ ___ ___ ___ ___

Patient 6   ___ ___ ___ ___ ___ ___ ___ ___

Patient 7   ___ ___ ___ ___ ___ ___ ___ ___

Patient 8   ___ ___ ___ ___ ___ ___ ___ ___

Patient 9   ___ ___ ___ ___ ___ ___ ___ ___

Patient 10   ___ ___ ___ ___ ___ ___ ___ ___

Patient 11   ___ ___ ___ ___ ___ ___ ___ ___

Patient 12   ___ ___ ___ ___ ___ ___ ___ ___

Patient 13   ___ ___ ___ ___ ___ ___ ___ ___

Patient 14   ___ ___ ___ ___ ___ ___ ___ ___

Patient 15   ___ ___ ___ ___ ___ ___ ___ ___

Electrocardiographic Diagnostic Coding Sheet

General Features
1. Normal ECG
2. Normal ECG, variant
3. Misplaced leads
4. Electrical alternans

Sinus Rhythms
5. Normal sinus
6. Sinus tachycardia
7. Sinus bradycardia
8. Sinus arrhythmia
9. Sinus pause or arrest

Atrial Rhythms
10. Premature atrial contractions (PAC)
11. Aberrant PAC
12. Ectopic atrial rhythm
13. Atrial tachycardia with AV block
14. Atrial fibrillation
15. Atrial flutter
16. Multifocal atrial tachycardia
17. Dual atrial rhythms

AV Junctional Rhythms
18. Premature junctional beats (PJB)
19. Aberrant PJB
20. Junctional beat or rhythm
21. AV junctional rhythm with retrograde atrial activation
22. Supraventricular tachycardia

Ventricular Rhythms
23. Premature ventricular contractions (PVC), unifocal
24. PVC, multifocal
25. PVC, couplets/triplets
26. PVC, R-on-T phenomenon
27. Ventricular tachycardia
28. Idioventricular rhythm
29. Ventricular fibrillation
30. Ventricular escape beat or rhythm
31. Ventricular fusion beat or rhythm
32. Ventricular capture beat during VT
33. Torsades de pointes

Pacemaker Rhythms
34. Fixed rate
35. Demand
36. Atrial pacing
37. Ventricular pacing
38. Dual chamber pacing
39. Failure to sense
40. Failure to capture

AV Conduction Abnormalities
41. 1° AV block
42. Wenckebach (Mobitz I) AV block
43. 2° AV block (Mobitz II)
44. Fixed 2° AV block, 2:1, 4:1, etc.
45. Complete heart block
46. Variable AV block
47. Preexcitation (WPW)

AV - VA Interactions
48. Fusion beat
49. Echo beat
50. AV dissociation
51. Isorhythmic AV dissociation

Intraventricular Conduction Abnormalities
52. Left axis
53. Right axis
54. Incomplete RBBB
55. Complete RBBB
56. Incomplete LBBB
57. Complete LBBB
58. Anterior hemiblock
59. Posterior hemiblock
60. Nonspecific IVCD
61. Arrhythmia related aberrancy
62. Intermittent IVCD/BBB

Chamber Enlargement
63. Left atrial enlargement
64. Right atrial enlargement
65. Bi-atrial enlargement
66. LVH - voltage
67. LVH - voltage plus repolarization changes
68. RVH
69. Biventricular hypertrophy

Myocardial Infarction

Recent/Acute
70. Anteroseptal
71. Anterior
72. Lateral
73. Inferior
74. Posterior

Old/Uncertain Age
75. Anteroseptal
76. Anterior
77. Lateral
78. Inferior
79. Posterior

Repolarization Changes
80. Possible LV aneurysm
81. Non-Q wave infarction
82. Early repolarization
83. Persistent juvenile T wave
84. ST-T wave changes of acute injury
85. ST-T wave changes of acute ischemia
86. ST-T wave changes of hypertrophy or altered intraventricular conduction (secondary repolarization changes)
87. ST-T wave changes of pericarditis
88. ST changes due to digitalis effect
89. Nonspecific ST-T wave changes
90. Postectopic T wave changes
91. Peaked T waves
92. Prolonged QT interval
93. Prominent U waves

Clinical Problems
94. Coronary artery disease
95. Congenital heart disease
96. Mitral valve disease
97. Hyperkalemia
98. Hypokalemia
99. Hypercalcemia
100. Hypocalcemia
101. Digitalis toxicity
102. CNS event
103. Motion artifact
104. Dextrocardia
105. Cardiac tamponade
106. Cardiac transplant
107. Chronic lung disease

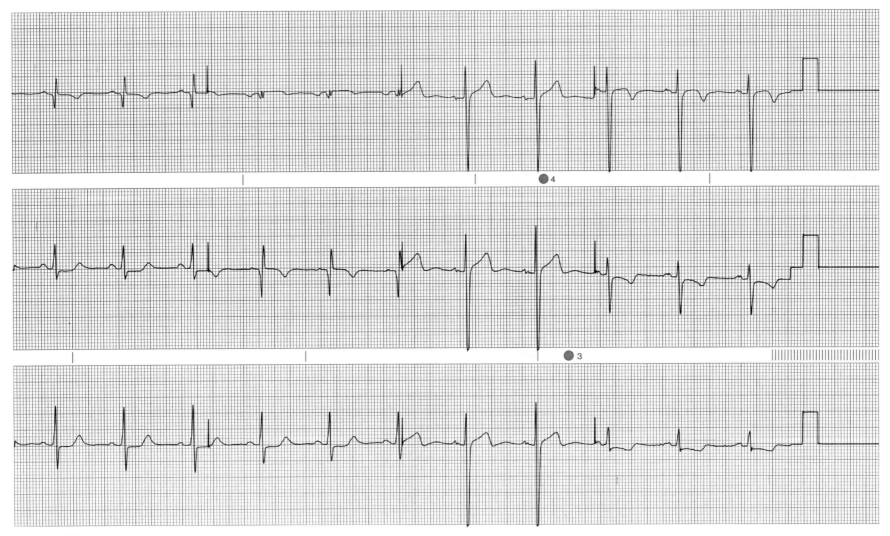

Exercise VII, Patient 1

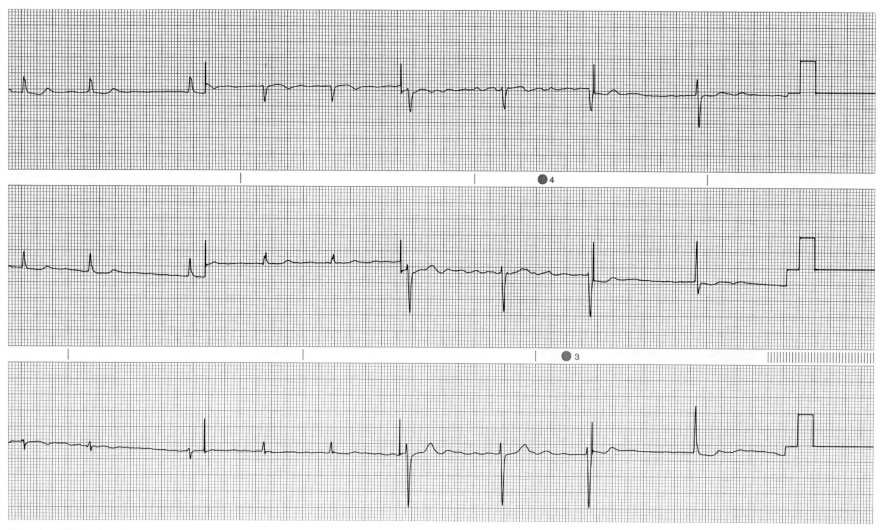

Exercise VII, Patient 2

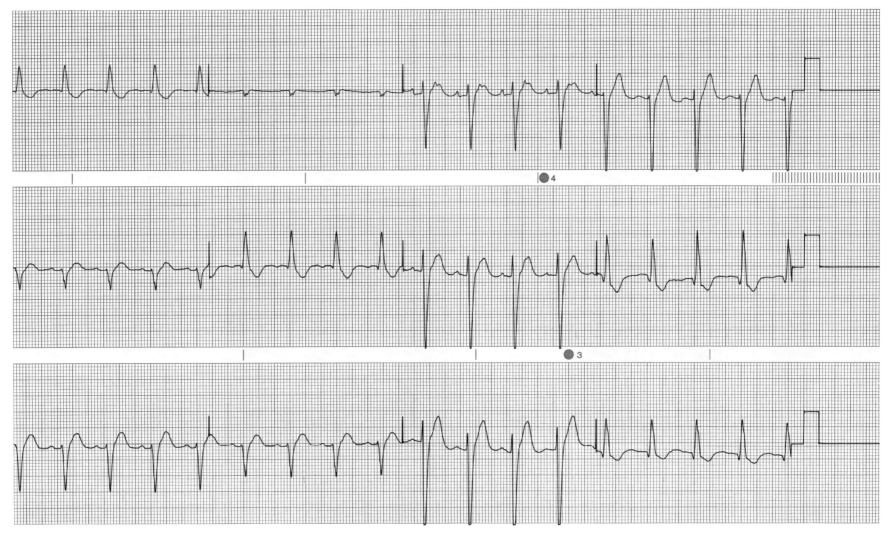

Exercise VII, Patient 3

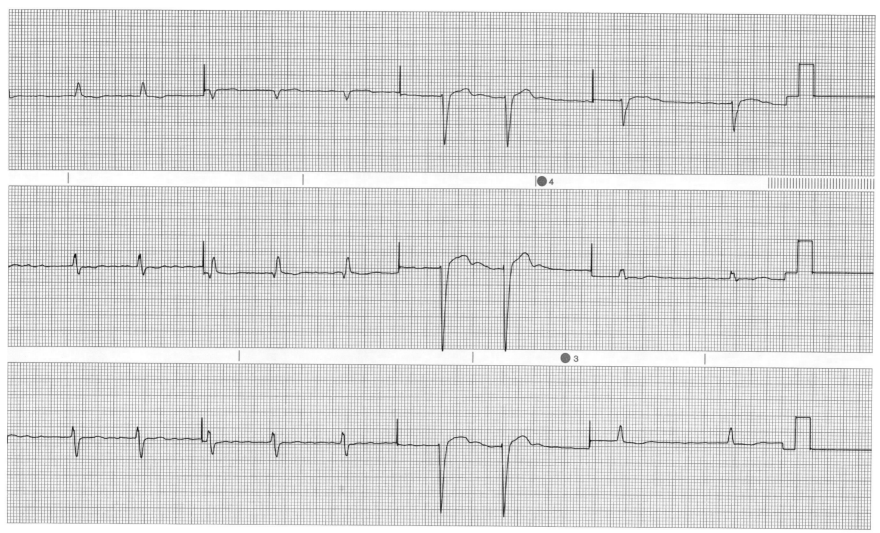

Exercise VII, Patient 4

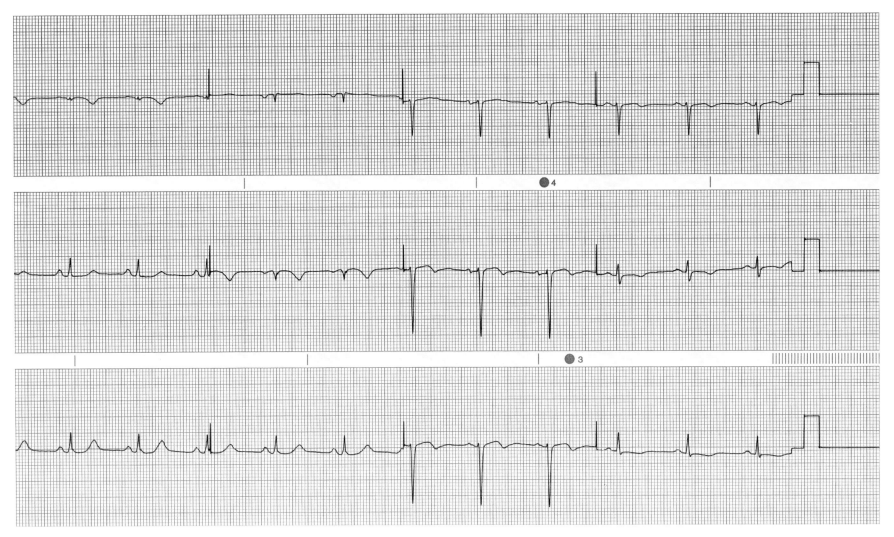

Exercise VII, Patient 5

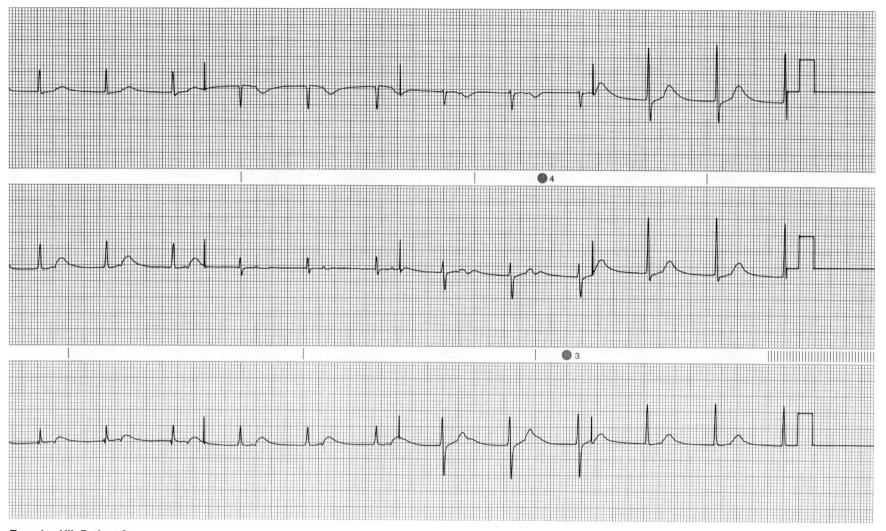

Exercise VII, Patient 6

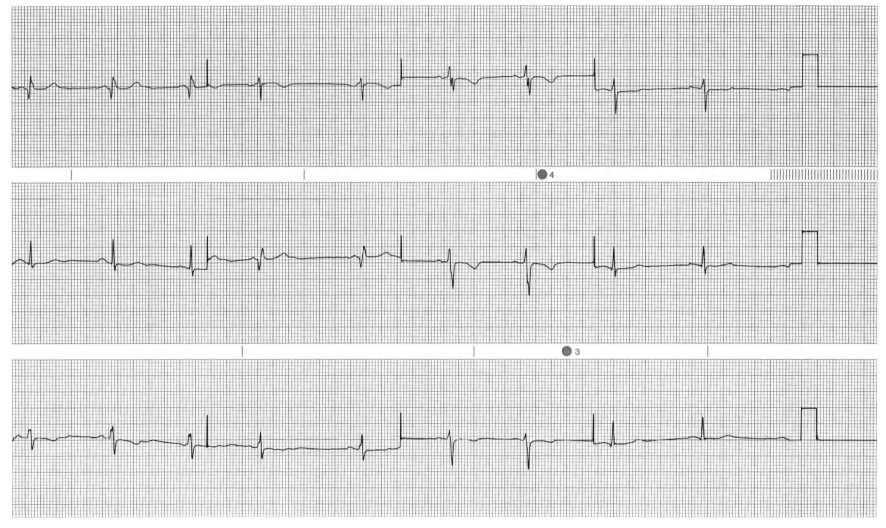

Exercise VII, Patient 7

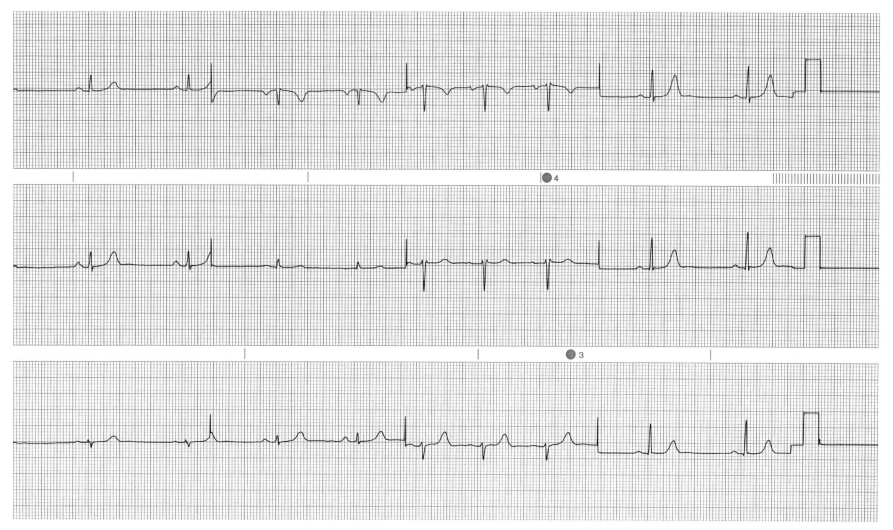

Exercise VII, Patient 8

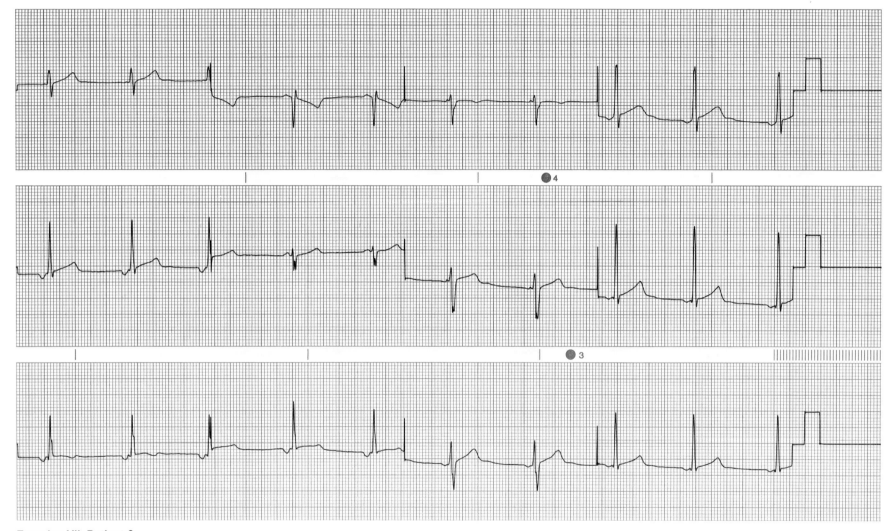

Exercise VII, Patient 9

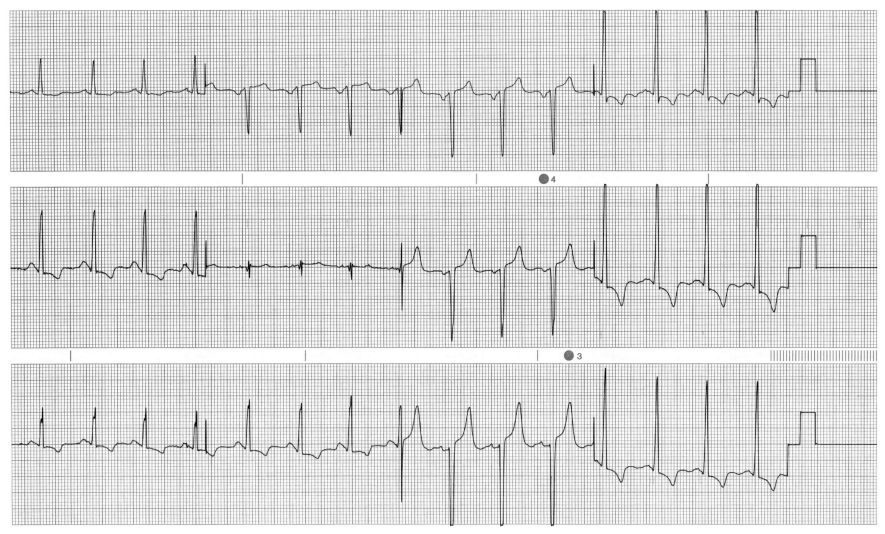

Exercise VII, Patient 10

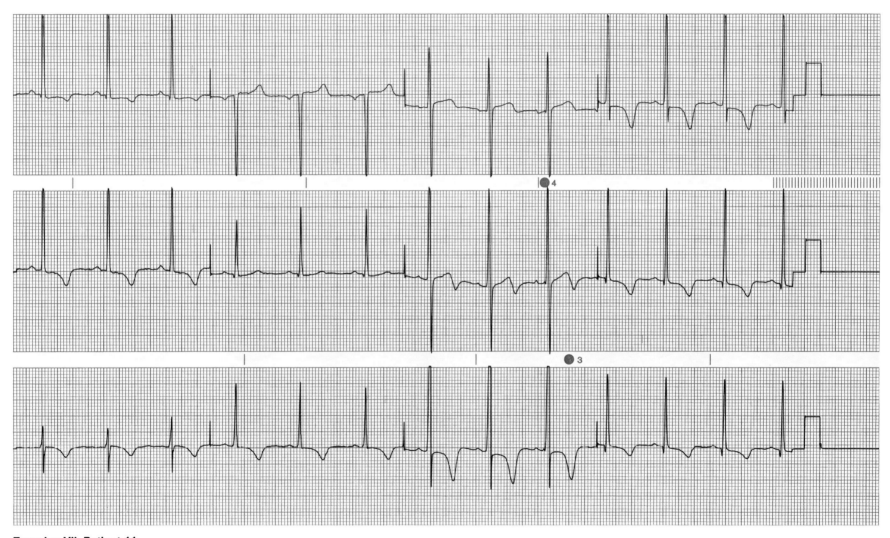

Exercise VII, Patient 11

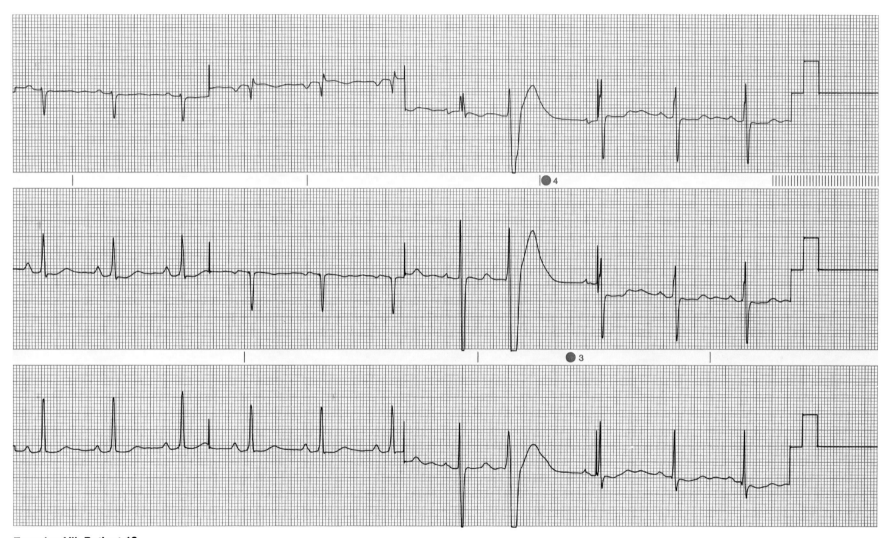

Exercise VII, Patient 12

Exercise VII, Patient 13

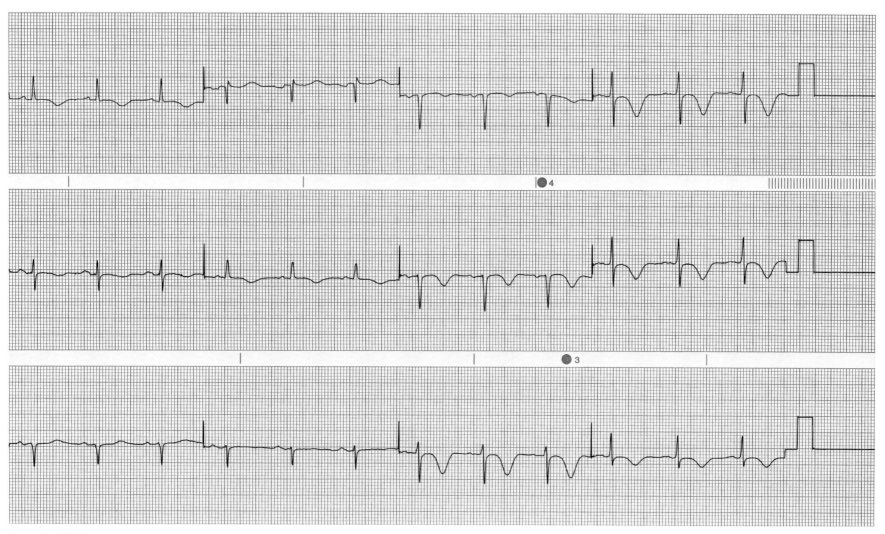

Exercise VII, Patient 14

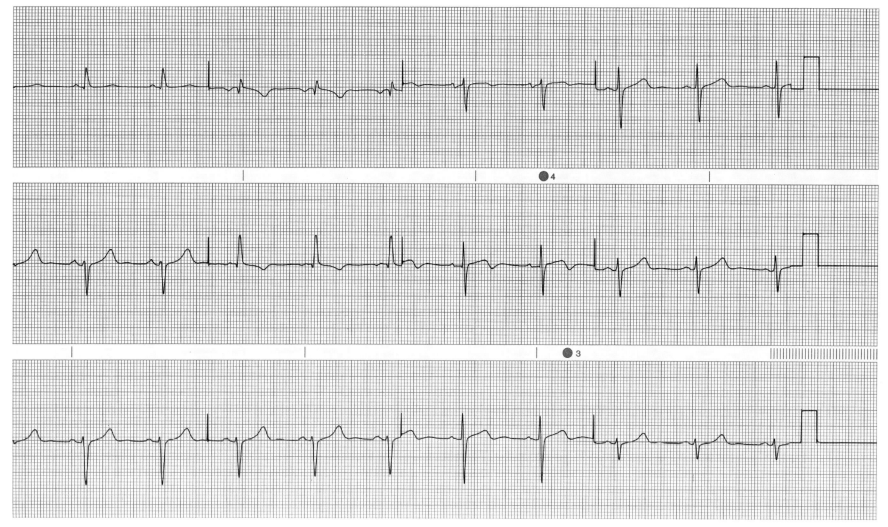

Exercise VII, Patient 15

1. This electrocardiogram shows a sinus rhythm with a high lateral infarction. There are Q waves in leads I and aV$_L$, and there is R wave regression from V$_3$ to V$_4$. These are associated with symmetric T wave inversions. Coded 5, 77, and 94.
2. This shows atrial fibrillation with digitalis effect. There is ST segment scooping in the lateral precordial leads and in leads I, II, and aV$_L$. The QT interval is relatively short. Coded 14 and 88.
3. This patient has atrial tachycardia with 2:1 block. There is left axis deviation and a small Q wave in lead aV$_L$ with secondary T wave changes, which might suggest an anterior hemiblock. The QRS complex is >120 milliseconds, however, so this would be better coded as intraventricular delay and left axis deviation. There is R wave regression in leads V$_1$ to V$_4$ and a broad Q wave in lead V$_5$, suggesting anterior infarct. Atrial tachycardia with block can be a digitalis toxic rhythm. Coded 13, 52, 60, 76, 86, and 94 (also possibly 101).
4. This electrocardiogram shows slow atrial fibrillation with an intraventricular delay and an anterolateral infarct. There are poor R wave progression and a relatively broad Q wave in lead aV$_L$. Coded 14, 60, 76, 77, 86, and 94.
5. This patient has a sinus rhythm and an anterolateral infarction. This is another example of poor R wave progression caused by infarct. Poor R wave progression with these T wave changes is enough to establish anterior infarction. The broad Q and T wave changes in lead aV$_L$, and to some extent in

lead I, also support this. Coded 5, 76, 77, and 94.
6. This electrocardiogram is normal except for the atypical location and axis of the P waves. This is a nodal rhythm with retrograde activation of the atria. This is from the same patient in Exercise II, patient 3, a month before her cerebral hemorrhage. Coded 21.
7. This patient has an old anterolateral infarct and nonspecific repolarization changes. There is R wave regression in leads V$_2$ to V$_3$ and deep Q waves in leads I and aV$_L$. Coded 7, 76, 77, 89, and 94.
8. This patient has a variable RR interval. All beats are preceded by normal P waves, however. This is an example of a sinus rhythm with a sinus arrhythmia. Coded 1, 7, and 8.
9. This is an example of a low atrial rhythm with inverted P waves in leads II and III. There is minimal ST segment elevation, consistent with early repolarization. This was a healthy young man. Coded 12 and 82.
10. This patient has a sinus rhythm, left atrial enlargement, and left ventricular hypertrophy. Left atrial enlargement is suggested by the broad P wave in lead II and the broadly negative P-terminal forces in lead V$_1$. Voltage is obviously prominent, and there are typical ST-T wave changes of ventricular strain in the lateral precordial and inferior leads. Coded 5, 63, 67, and 86. This is an example of poor R wave progression in the anterior precordial leads caused by ventricular hypertrophy rather than infarction.
11. This electrocardiogram shows a sinus rhythm with left ventricular hypertrophy. This patient with hypertrophic cardiomyop-

athy had generalized ventricular thickening but no intracardiac gradient. Hypertrophic cardiomyopathy is suggested by the prominence of the R waves in leads V$_1$ and V$_2$, counterclockwise rotation despite ventricular hypertrophy, and the mid precordial T wave changes. Coded 5 and 67.
12. This electrocardiogram shows a sinus rhythm with premature ventricular contractions (PVCs). Right ventricular hypertrophy is evidenced by the prominent voltage in lead V$_1$ with secondary T wave changes and marked right axis deviation. The lateral ST-T wave changes with prominent U waves are also consistent with hypokalemia. Coded 5, 23, 53, 68, 93, and 98.
13. This patient has a sinus rhythm with sinus arrhythmia and preexcitation. Coded 5, 8, and 47.
14. This electrocardiogram shows prominent symmetric T wave inversion, especially in the mid precordial leads but also generally throughout the electrocardiogram. The generalized nature of the T wave changes, their symmetry, and the prolonged QT interval suggest a recent intracerebral event, although a non–Q wave infarct is possible. Coded 5, 52, 92, and 102 (or possibly 81 and 94).
15. This patient has a sinus rhythm with anterior hemiblock. There is marked left axis deviation with a predominantly negative vector in lead II. The QRS duration is <120 milliseconds, and the QRS pattern in lead aV$_L$ shows a Q wave, a delay in activation, and secondary repolarization abnormalities. Coded 5, 58, and 86.

Exercise VIII

ANSWER SHEET
Exercise VIII

Patient 1   ___ ___ ___ ___ ___ ___ ___

Patient 2   ___ ___ ___ ___ ___ ___ ___

Patient 3   ___ ___ ___ ___ ___ ___ ___

Patient 4   ___ ___ ___ ___ ___ ___ ___

Patient 5   ___ ___ ___ ___ ___ ___ ___

Patient 6   ___ ___ ___ ___ ___ ___ ___

Patient 7   ___ ___ ___ ___ ___ ___ ___

Patient 8   ___ ___ ___ ___ ___ ___ ___

Patient 9   ___ ___ ___ ___ ___ ___ ___

Patient 10   ___ ___ ___ ___ ___ ___ ___

Patient 11   ___ ___ ___ ___ ___ ___ ___

Patient 12   ___ ___ ___ ___ ___ ___ ___

Patient 13   ___ ___ ___ ___ ___ ___ ___

Patient 14   ___ ___ ___ ___ ___ ___ ___

Patient 15   ___ ___ ___ ___ ___ ___ ___

Electrocardiographic Diagnostic Coding Sheet

General Features
1. Normal ECG
2. Normal ECG, variant
3. Misplaced leads
4. Electrical alternans

Sinus Rhythms
5. Normal sinus
6. Sinus tachycardia
7. Sinus bradycardia
8. Sinus arrhythmia
9. Sinus pause or arrest

Atrial Rhythms
10. Premature atrial contractions (PAC)
11. Aberrant PAC
12. Ectopic atrial rhythm
13. Atrial tachycardia with AV block
14. Atrial fibrillation
15. Atrial flutter
16. Multifocal atrial tachycardia
17. Dual atrial rhythms

AV Junctional Rhythms
18. Premature junctional beats (PJB)
19. Aberrant PJB
20. Junctional beat or rhythm
21. AV junctional rhythm with retrograde atrial activation
22. Supraventricular tachycardia

Ventricular Rhythms
23. Premature ventricular contractions (PVC), unifocal
24. PVC, multifocal
25. PVC, couplets/triplets
26. PVC, R-on-T phenomenon
27. Ventricular tachycardia
28. Idioventricular rhythm
29. Ventricular fibrillation
30. Ventricular escape beat or rhythm
31. Ventricular fusion beat or rhythm
32. Ventricular capture beat during VT
33. Torsades de pointes

Pacemaker Rhythms
34. Fixed rate
35. Demand
36. Atrial pacing
37. Ventricular pacing
38. Dual chamber pacing
39. Failure to sense
40. Failure to capture

AV Conduction Abnormalities
41. 1° AV block
42. Wenckebach (Mobitz I) AV block
43. 2° AV block (Mobitz II)
44. Fixed 2° AV block, 2:1, 4:1, etc.
45. Complete heart block
46. Variable AV block
47. Preexcitation (WPW)

AV - VA Interactions
48. Fusion beat
49. Echo beat
50. AV dissociation
51. Isorhythmic AV dissociation

Intraventricular Conduction Abnormalities
52. Left axis
53. Right axis
54. Incomplete RBBB
55. Complete RBBB
56. Incomplete LBBB
57. Complete LBBB
58. Anterior hemiblock
59. Posterior hemiblock
60. Nonspecific IVCD
61. Arrhythmia related aberrancy
62. Intermittent IVCD/BBB

Chamber Enlargement
63. Left atrial enlargement
64. Right atrial enlargement
65. Bi-atrial enlargement
66. LVH - voltage
67. LVH - voltage plus repolarization changes
68. RVH
69. Biventricular hypertrophy

Myocardial Infarction
Recent/Acute
70. Anteroseptal
71. Anterior
72. Lateral
73. Inferior
74. Posterior

Old/Uncertain Age
75. Anteroseptal
76. Anterior
77. Lateral
78. Inferior
79. Posterior

Repolarization Changes
80. Possible LV aneurysm
81. Non-Q wave infarction
82. Early repolarization
83. Persistent juvenile T wave
84. ST-T wave changes of acute injury
85. ST-T wave changes of acute ischemia
86. ST-T wave changes of hypertrophy or altered intraventricular conduction (secondary repolarization changes)
87. ST-T wave changes of pericarditis
88. ST changes due to digitalis effect
89. Nonspecific ST-T wave changes
90. Postectopic T wave changes
91. Peaked T waves
92. Prolonged QT interval
93. Prominent U waves

Clinical Problems
94. Coronary artery disease
95. Congenital heart disease
96. Mitral valve disease
97. Hyperkalemia
98. Hypokalemia
99. Hypercalcemia
100. Hypocalcemia
101. Digitalis toxicity
102. CNS event
103. Motion artifact
104. Dextrocardia
105. Cardiac tamponade
106. Cardiac transplant
107. Chronic lung disease

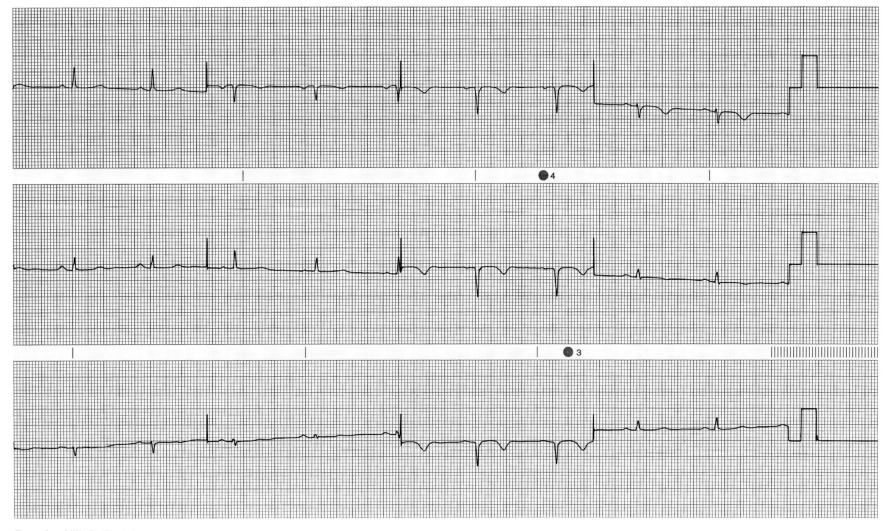

Exercise VIII, Patient 1

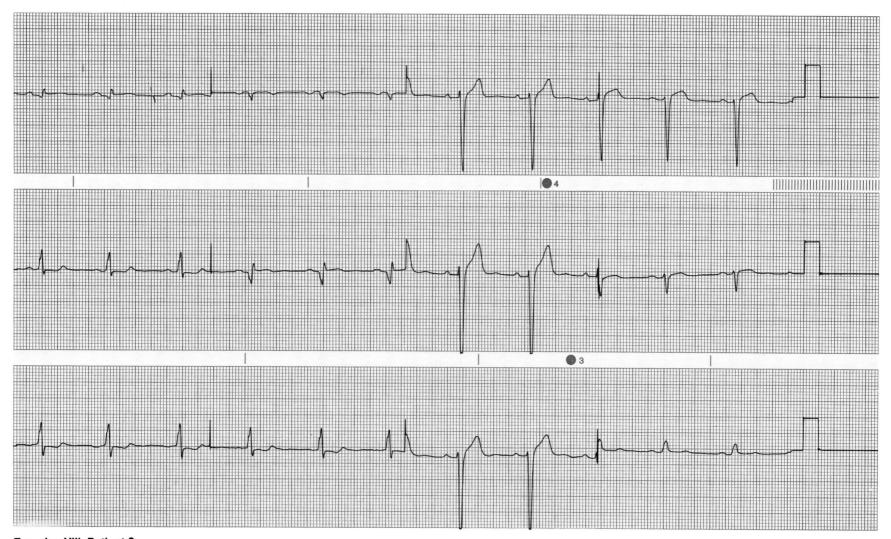

Exercise VIII, Patient 2

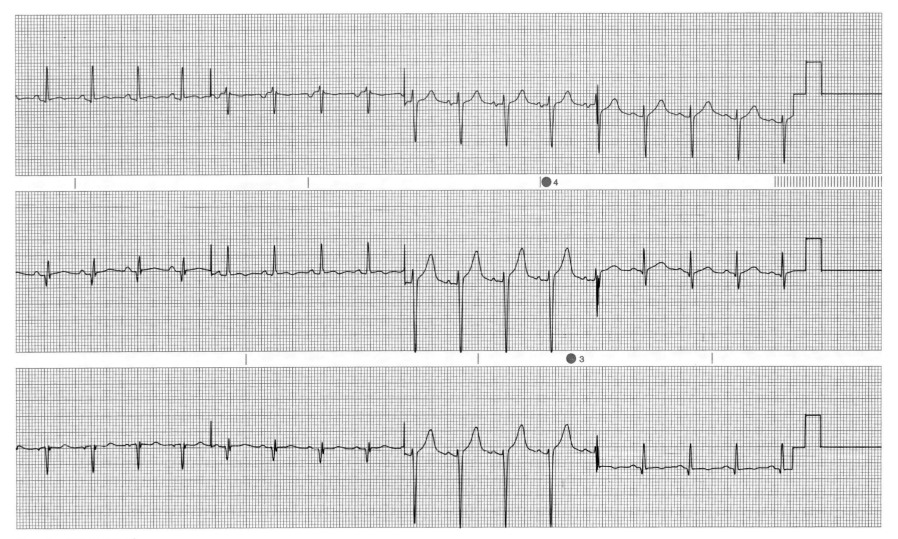

Exercise VIII, Patient 3

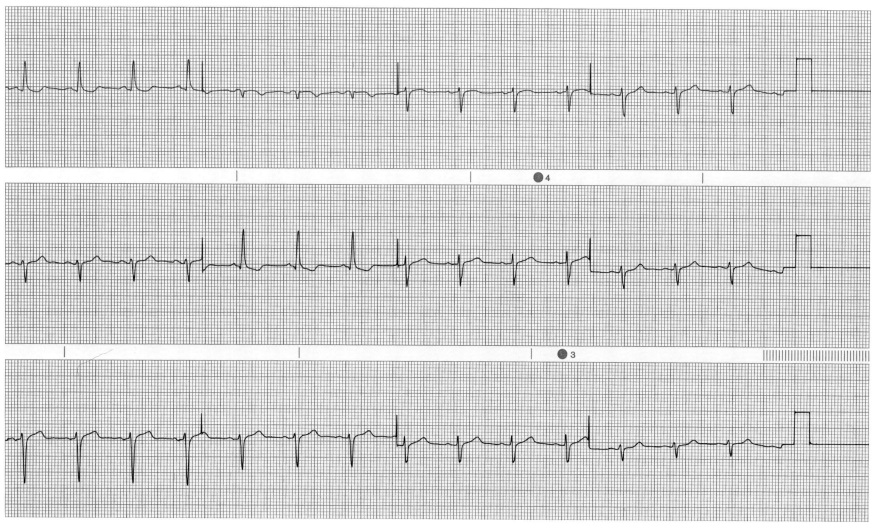

Exercise VIII, Patient 4

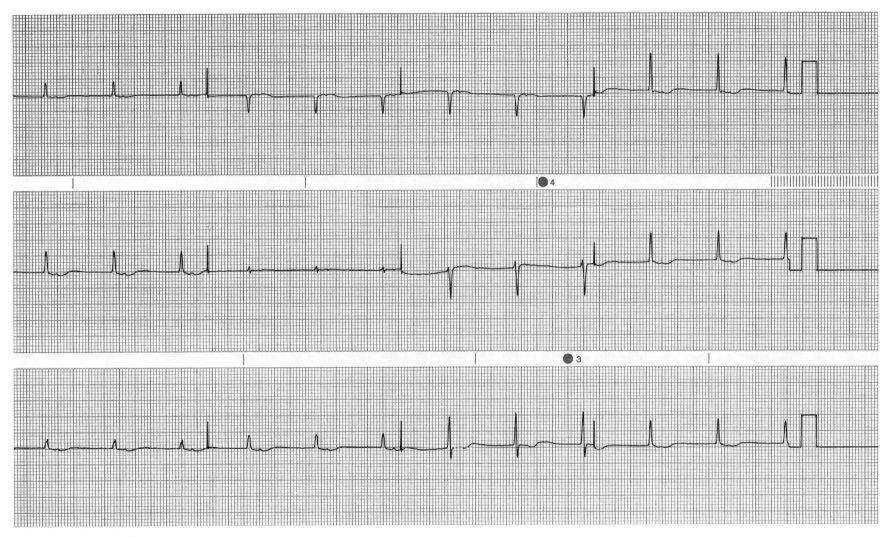

Exercise VIII, Patient 5

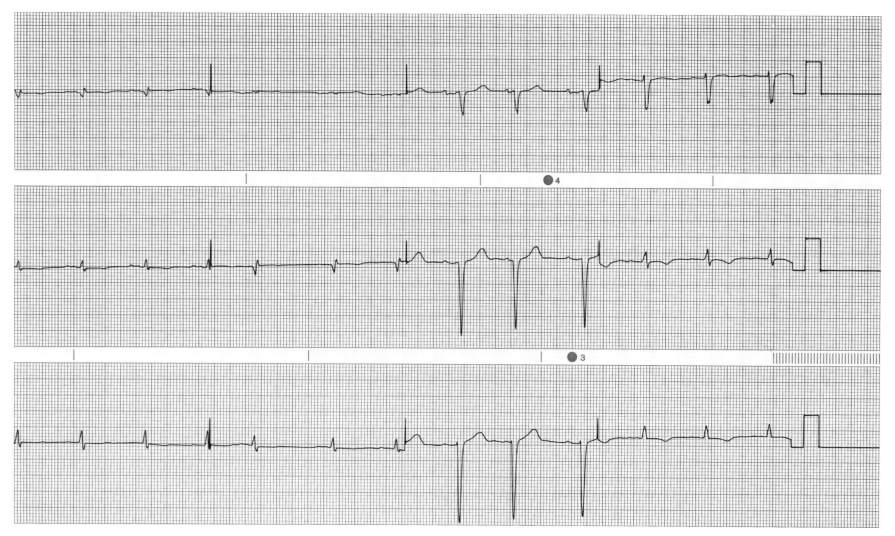

Exercise VIII, Patient 6

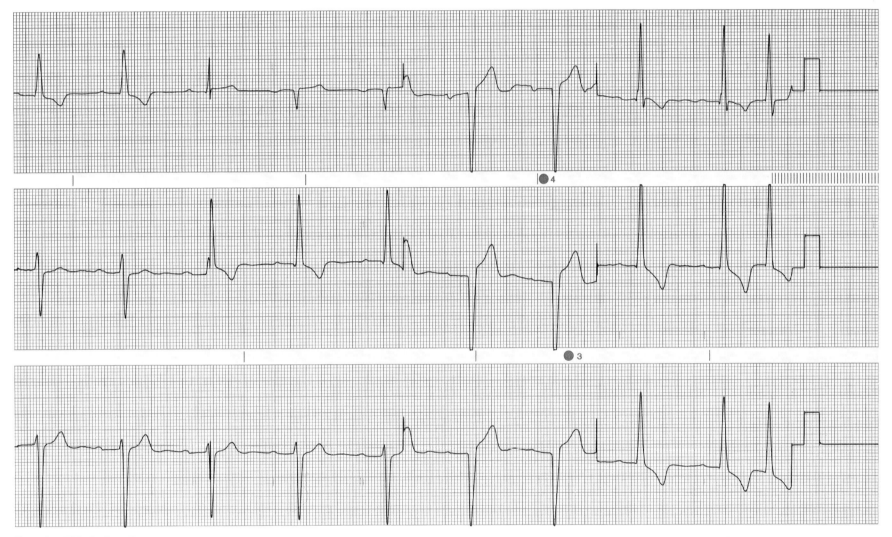

Exercise VIII, Patient 7

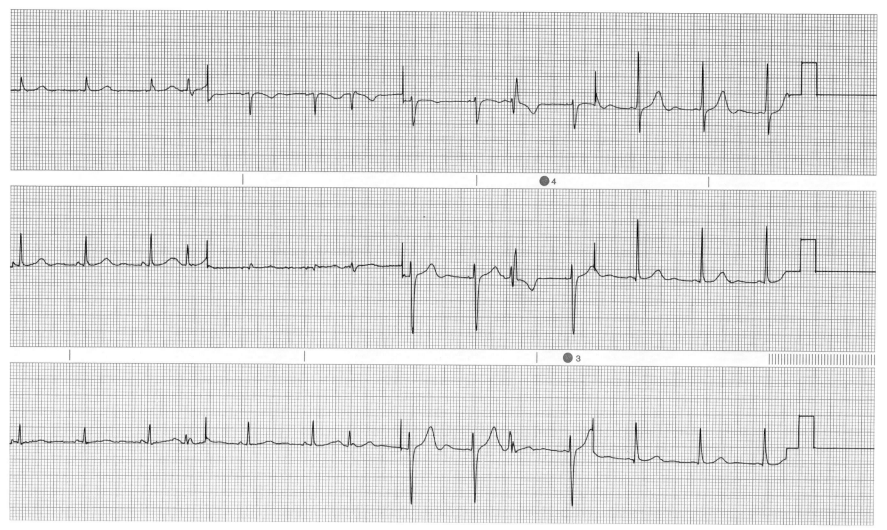

Exercise VIII, Patient 8

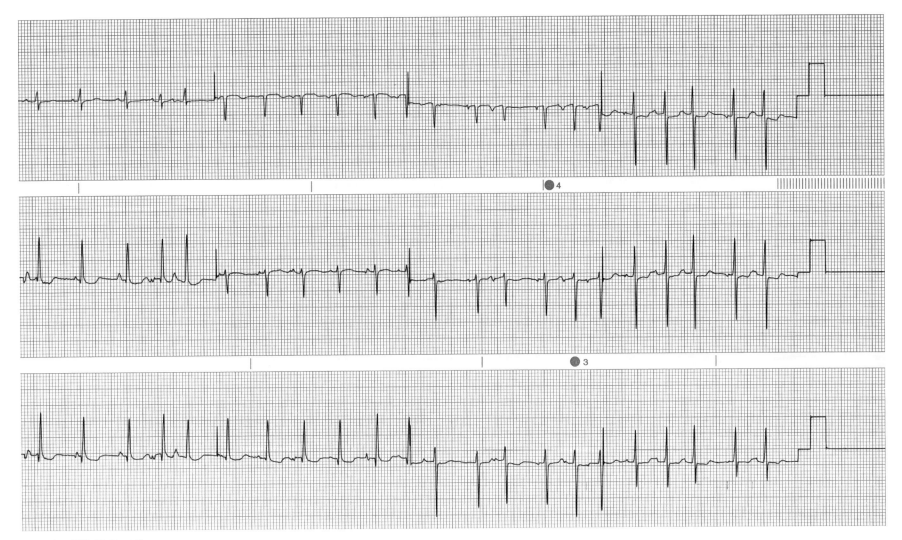

Exercise VIII, Patient 9

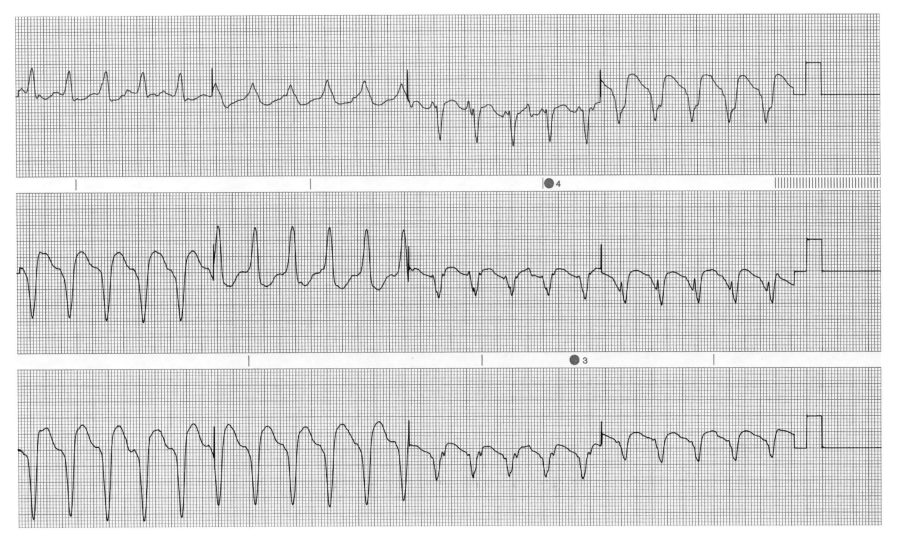

Exercise VIII, Patient 10

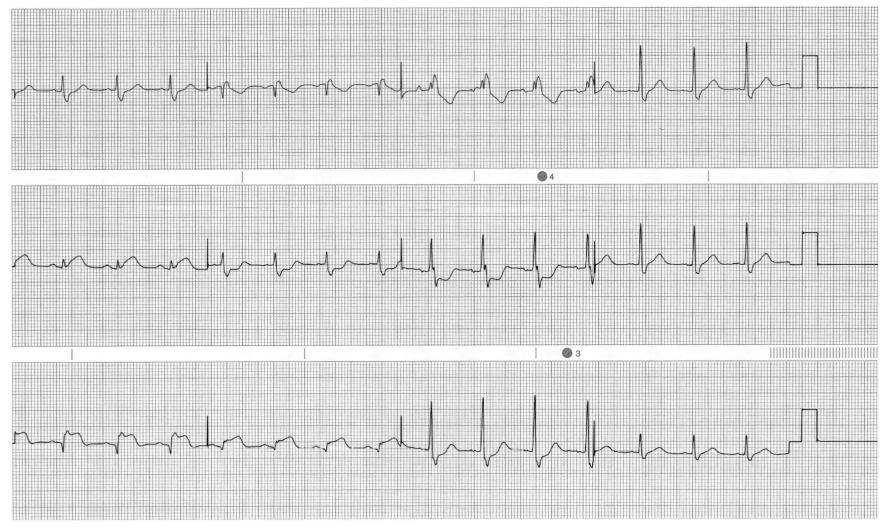

Exercise VIII, Patient 11

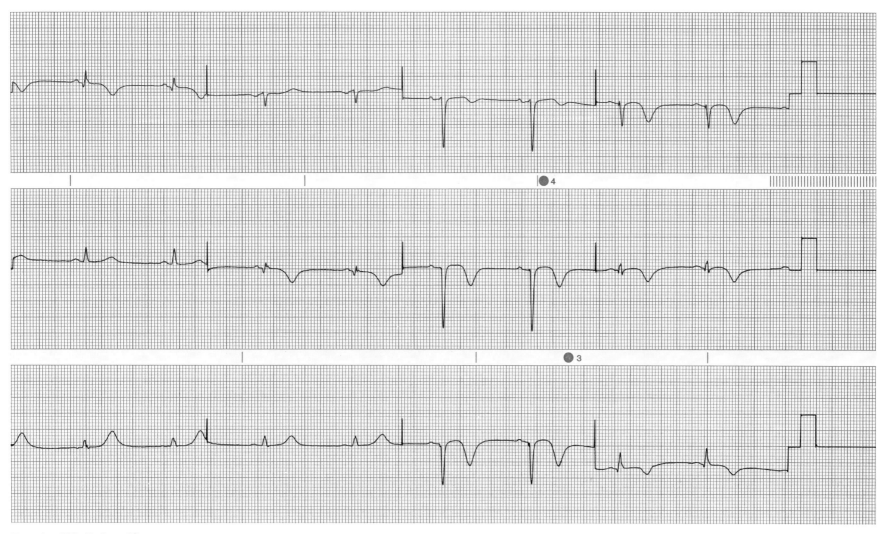

Exercise VIII, Patient 12

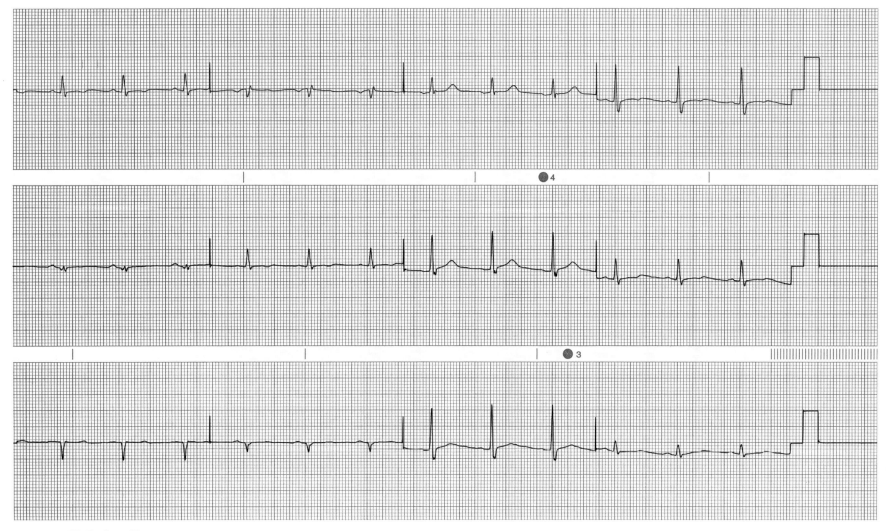

Exercise VIII, Patient 13

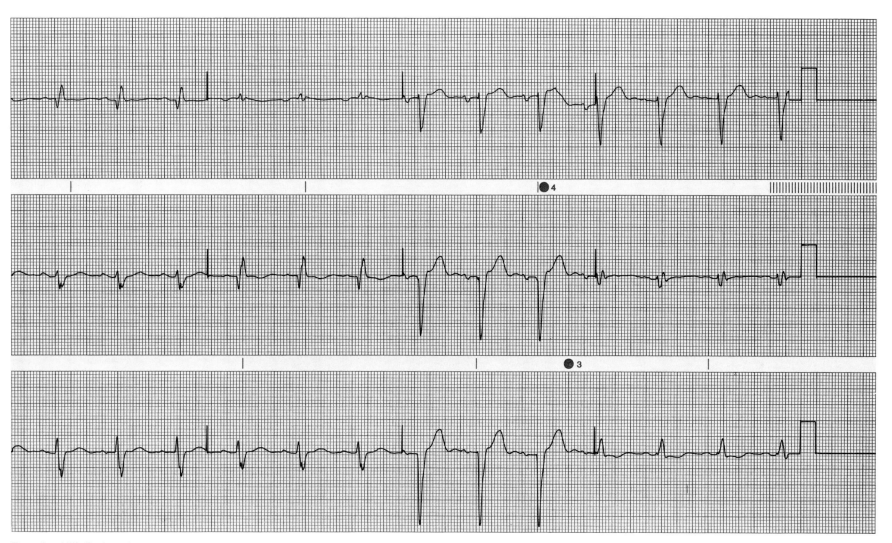

Exercise VIII, Patient 14

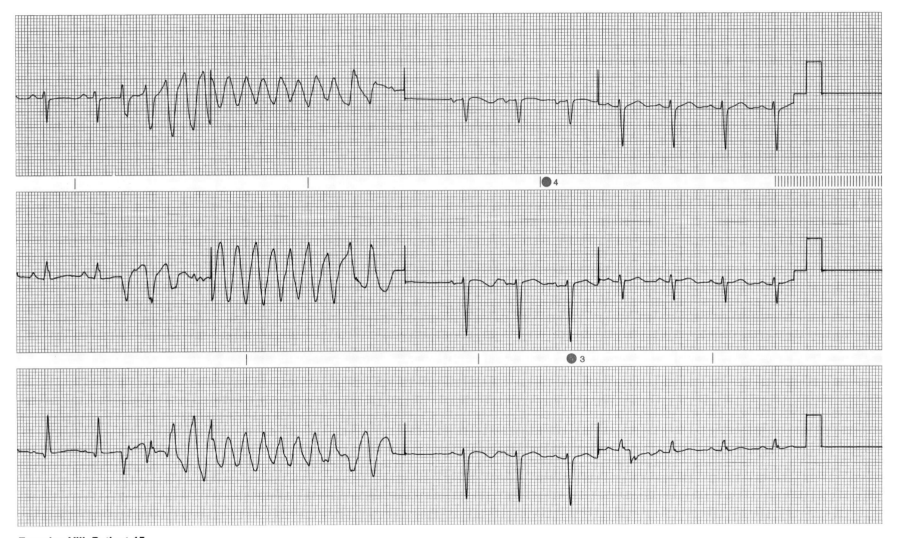

Exercise VIII, Patient 15

1. This electrocardiogram shows Q waves in leads V_1 to V_3, and T wave inversion in leads V_1 to V_4. This is an anteroseptal infarction of uncertain age. T waves like this can be seen in both recent and more established infarctions, so their presence does not help differentiate acuity of the event. Coded 7, 75, and 94.

2. This electrocardiogram shows R wave regression with Q waves in the lateral leads. This is an anterolateral infarct of either remote or uncertain age. Coded 5, 76, 77, and 94.

3. This is an inferior infarction with deep, wide Q waves in leads V_6, aV_F, and II. There is also R wave regression from leads V_2 and V_3 but normal-appearing T waves. R wave regression with normal-appearing T waves is an inconclusive sign for infarct. Coded 6, 78, and 94 (also possibly 76).

4. This is an anterior hemiblock. The axis is to the left, and lead aV_L shows a small Q wave, slight activation delay, and secondary repolarization changes. Coded 5, 58, and 86.

5. This electrocardiogram shows a junctional rhythm with retrograde P waves. There are nonspecific repolarization abnormalities. Coded 21 and 89.

6. This electrocardiogram shows an anterolateral infarction. There is poor R wave progression across the precordium associated with broad Q waves in leads I and aV_L. In the third panel there is a premature atrial contraction as well as nonspecific repolarization changes laterally. Coded 5, 10, 76, 77, 89, and 94.

7. This shows a sinus rhythm with a first-degree AV block. The P waves are broadly negative in lead V_1, consistent with left atrial enlargement. The QRS complex is prolonged >120 milliseconds with small Q waves in leads I and V_6, indicating a nonspecific intraventricular delay rather than a complete left bundle branch block. Voltage and repolarization changes in aV_L and in the lateral precordial leads suggest ventricular hypertrophy. There is left axis deviation as well as a premature junctional beat terminating the tracing. Leads V_1 to V_3 have Q waves suggesting anteroseptal infarction. This electrocardiogram should be coded as showing sinus bradycardia with a first-degree AV block, intraventricular delay, premature junctional contraction, left ventricular hypertrophy, left axis, and an old anteroseptal infarction. Coded 7, 18, 41, 52, 60, 67, 75, 86, and 94.

8. This electrocardiogram is normal but does show a premature atrial contraction with aberrancy. Coded 1, 5, and 11.

9. This electrocardiogram has a chaotic ventricular response. In the third panel, three separate atrial foci can be seen, suggesting a diagnosis of multifocal atrial tachycardia. In addition, the R : S ratio is <1 in lead V_5, raising the possibility of right ventricular hypertrophy. This is a rhythm seen with chronic lung disease, usually decompensated. Coded 16, 68, 89, and 107.

10. This electrocardiogram shows a wide complex tachycardia. It has anterior concordance, a sinus rhythm, but AV dissociation, indicating ventricular tachycardia. Coded 5, 27, and 50.

11. This electrocardiogram shows a sinus rhythm with a complete right bundle branch block and an acute inferior myocardial infarction. The right bundle branch block is established by the wide R' in lead V_1 and the broad terminal S in lead V_6. The infarct is diagnosed by the presence of ST segment elevation in leads III and aV_F, the symmetric T wave in lead II, and the horizontal ST segment depression in leads aV_L and V_2, which are reciprocal changes of the acute infarct. Coded 5, 55, 73, 84, and 94.

12. This shows symmetric T wave inversion. The depth of the T waves is relatively great. The QT interval is not particularly prolonged. In addition, there is R wave regression leading to Q waves in leads V_2, V_3, and V_4 and a relatively broad and deep Q wave in lead aV_L. Although this might indicate an acute intracerebral episode, the Q waves suggest rather that these T wave changes are related to anterolateral infarction. Coded 7, 76, 77, and 94.

13. This is an inferoposterior infarction. The patient has a sinus rhythm and broad Q waves in leads aV_F, II, and III. There are also prominent R waves with upright T waves in leads V_1 and V_2. Coded 5, 78, 79, and 94.

14. This patient has an anterolateral infarction with R wave regression, Q waves in leads V_2 and V_3, and broad Q waves in leads I and aV_L. In addition, there is a marked left axis. This should not be coded as a hemiblock because of the width of the QRS complex (>120 milliseconds). There are nonspecific lateral ST-T wave changes. This is not a complete left bundle branch block because of the Q wave in lead I. Coded 5, 52, 60, 76, 77, 89, and 94.

15. This electrocardiogram shows sinus rhythm with a burst of ventricular tachycardia. There is probable right ventricular hypertrophy as well as transient postectopic T wave changes. Right ventricular hypertrophy is suggested by the right axis and reversal of the R : S ratio with S >R in lead V_5. The posttachycardia T wave changes are seen in the first beat (in leads V_1 to V_3) following the burst of ventricular tachycardia as a greater T wave inversion than in the subsequent two beats. Coded 5, 27, 53, 68, 86, and 90.

Exercise IX

ANSWER SHEET
Exercise IX

Patient 1   —— —— —— —— —— —— —— ——

Patient 2   —— —— —— —— —— —— —— ——

Patient 3   —— —— —— —— —— —— —— ——

Patient 4   —— —— —— —— —— —— —— ——

Patient 5   —— —— —— —— —— —— —— ——

Patient 6   —— —— —— —— —— —— —— ——

Patient 7   —— —— —— —— —— —— —— ——

Patient 8   —— —— —— —— —— —— —— ——

Patient 9   —— —— —— —— —— —— —— ——

Patient 10   —— —— —— —— —— —— —— ——

Patient 11   —— —— —— —— —— —— —— ——

Patient 12   —— —— —— —— —— —— —— ——

Patient 13   —— —— —— —— —— —— —— ——

Patient 14   —— —— —— —— —— —— —— ——

Patient 15   —— —— —— —— —— —— —— ——

Electrocardiographic Diagnostic Coding Sheet

General Features
1. Normal ECG
2. Normal ECG, variant
3. Misplaced leads
4. Electrical alternans

Sinus Rhythms
5. Normal sinus
6. Sinus tachycardia
7. Sinus bradycardia
8. Sinus arrhythmia
9. Sinus pause or arrest

Atrial Rhythms
10. Premature atrial contractions (PAC)
11. Aberrant PAC
12. Ectopic atrial rhythm
13. Atrial tachycardia with AV block
14. Atrial fibrillation
15. Atrial flutter
16. Multifocal atrial tachycardia
17. Dual atrial rhythms

AV Junctional Rhythms
18. Premature junctional beats (PJB)
19. Aberrant PJB
20. Junctional beat or rhythm
21. AV junctional rhythm with retrograde atrial activation
22. Supraventricular tachycardia

Ventricular Rhythms
23. Premature ventricular contractions (PVC), unifocal
24. PVC, multifocal
25. PVC, couplets/triplets
26. PVC, R-on-T
27. Ventricular tachycardia
28. Idioventricular rhythm
29. Ventricular fibrillation
30. Ventricular escape beat or rhythm
31. Ventricular fusion beat or rhythm
32. Ventricular capture beat during VT
33. Torsades de pointes

Pacemaker Rhythms
34. Fixed rate
35. Demand
36. Atrial pacing
37. Ventricular pacing
38. Dual chamber pacing
39. Failure to sense
40. Failure to capture

AV Conduction Abnormalities
41. 1° AV block
42. Wenckebach (Mobitz I) AV block
43. 2° AV block (Mobitz II)
44. Fixed 2° AV block, 2:1, 4:1, etc.
45. Complete heart block
46. Variable AV block
47. Preexcitation (WPW)

AV - VA Interactions
48. Fusion beat
49. Echo beat
50. AV dissociation
51. Isorhythmic AV dissociation

Intraventricular Conduction Abnormalities
52. Left axis
53. Right axis
54. Incomplete RBBB
55. Complete RBBB
56. Incomplete LBBB
57. Complete LBBB
58. Anterior hemiblock
59. Posterior hemiblock
60. Nonspecific IVCD
61. Arrhythmia related aberrancy
62. Intermittent IVCD/BBB

Chamber Enlargement
63. Left atrial enlargement
64. Right atrial enlargement
65. Bi-atrial enlargement
66. LVH - voltage
67. LVH - voltage plus repolarization changes
68. RVH
69. Biventricular hypertrophy

Myocardial Infarction

Recent/Acute
70. Anteroseptal
71. Anterior
72. Lateral
73. Inferior
74. Posterior

Old/Uncertain Age
75. Anteroseptal
76. Anterior
77. Lateral
78. Inferior
79. Posterior

Repolarization Changes
80. Possible LV aneurysm
81. Non-Q wave infarction
82. Early repolarization
83. Persistent juvenile T wave
84. ST-T wave changes of acute injury
85. ST-T wave changes of acute ischemia
86. ST-T wave changes of hypertrophy or altered intraventricular conduction (secondary repolarization changes)
87. ST-T wave changes of pericarditis
88. ST changes due to digitalis effect
89. Nonspecific ST-T wave changes
90. Postectopic T wave changes
91. Peaked T waves
92. Prolonged QT interval
93. Prominent U waves

Clinical Problems
94. Coronary artery disease
95. Congenital heart disease
96. Mitral valve disease
97. Hyperkalemia
98. Hypokalemia
99. Hypercalcemia
100. Hypocalcemia
101. Digitalis toxicity
102. CNS event
103. Motion artifact
104. Dextrocardia
105. Cardiac tamponade
106. Cardiac transplant
107. Chronic lung disease

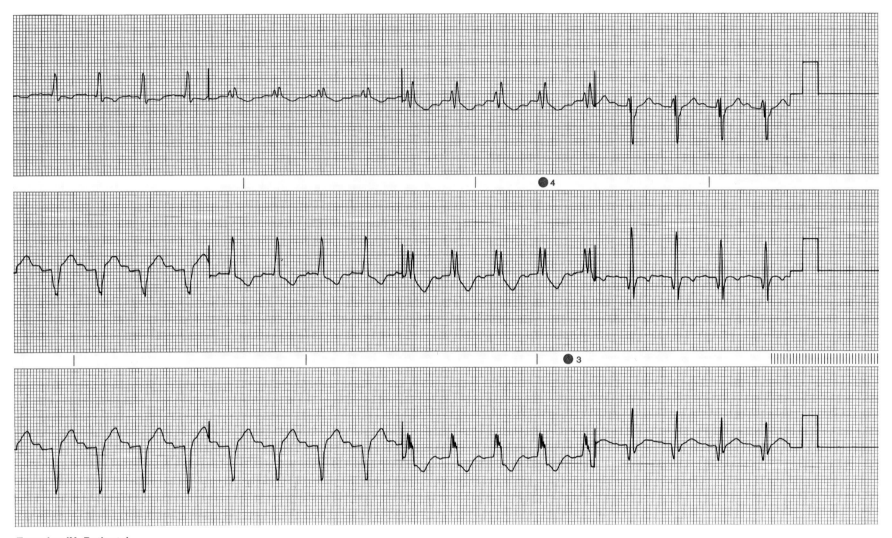

Exercise IX, Patient 1

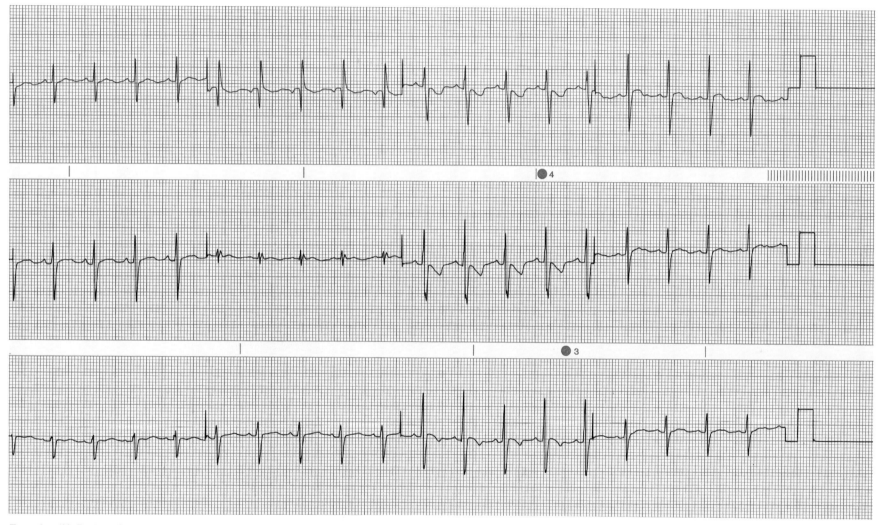

Exercise IX, Patient 2

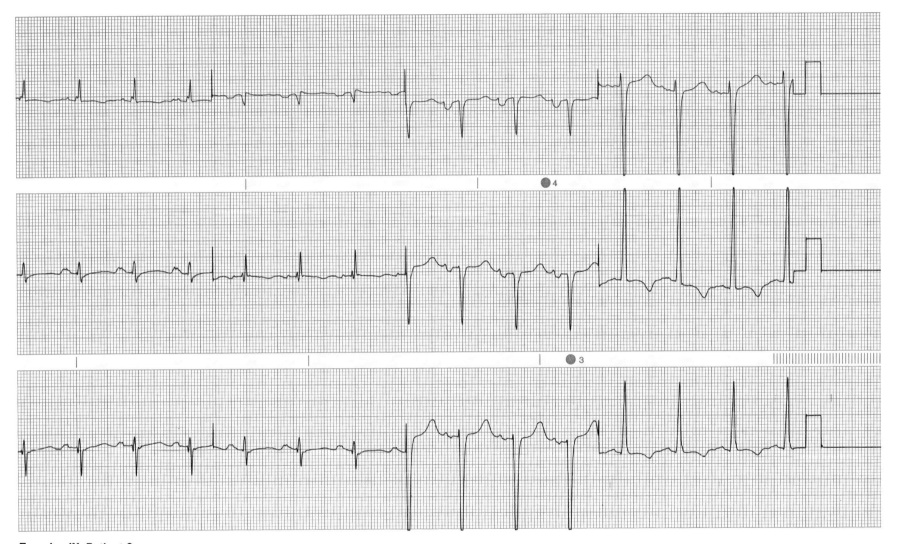

Exercise IX, Patient 3

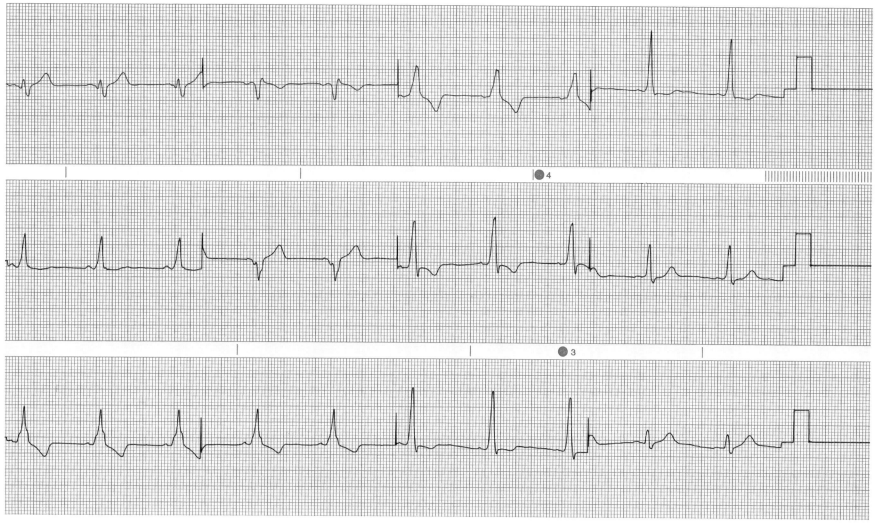

Exercise IX, Patient 4

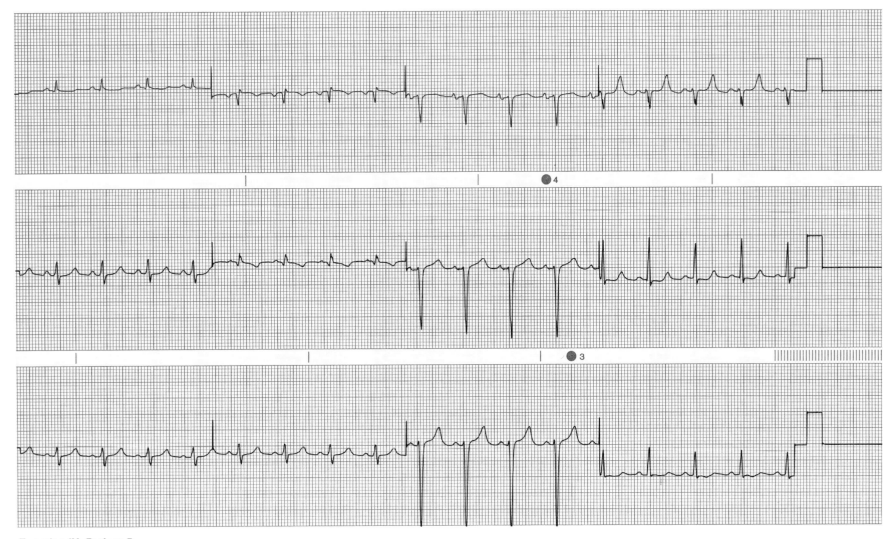

Exercise IX, Patient 5

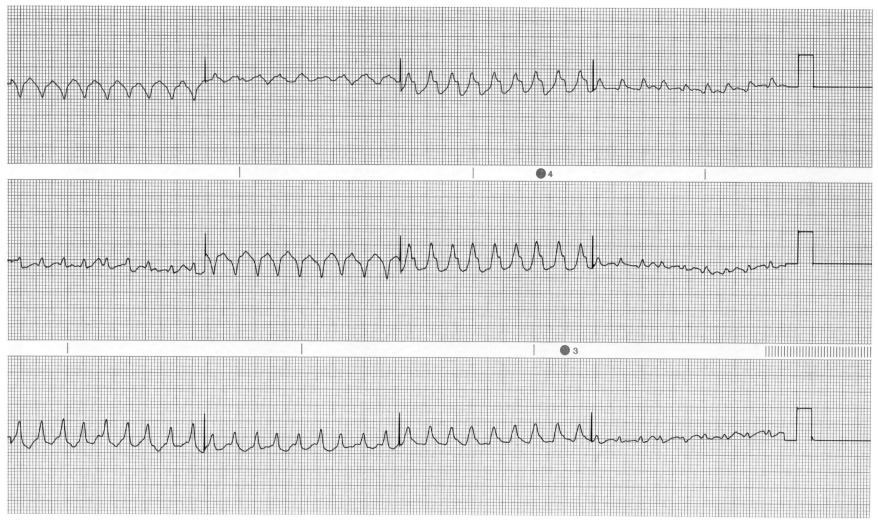

Exercise IX, Patient 6

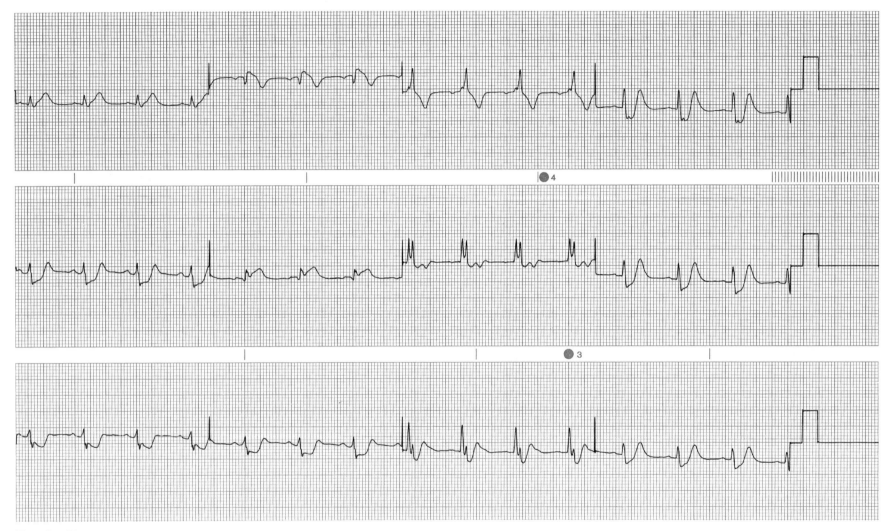

Exercise IX, Patient 7

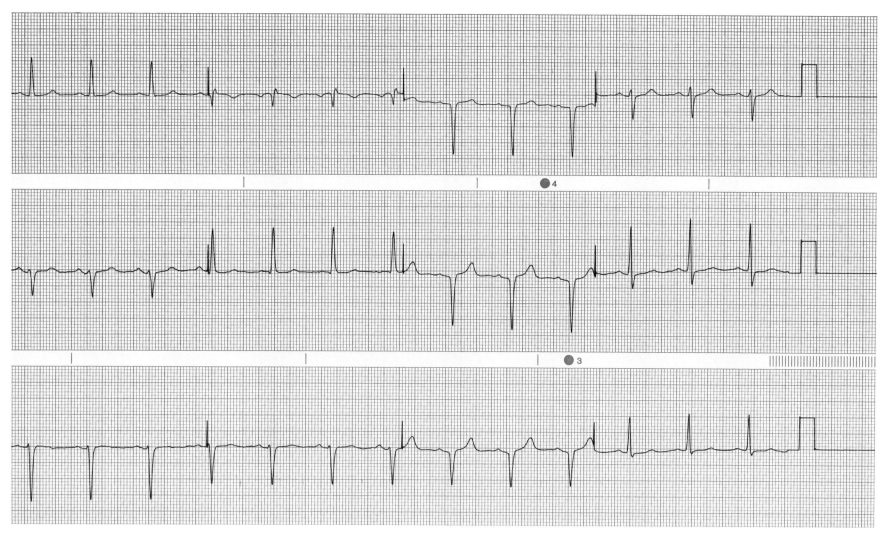

Exercise IX, Patient 8

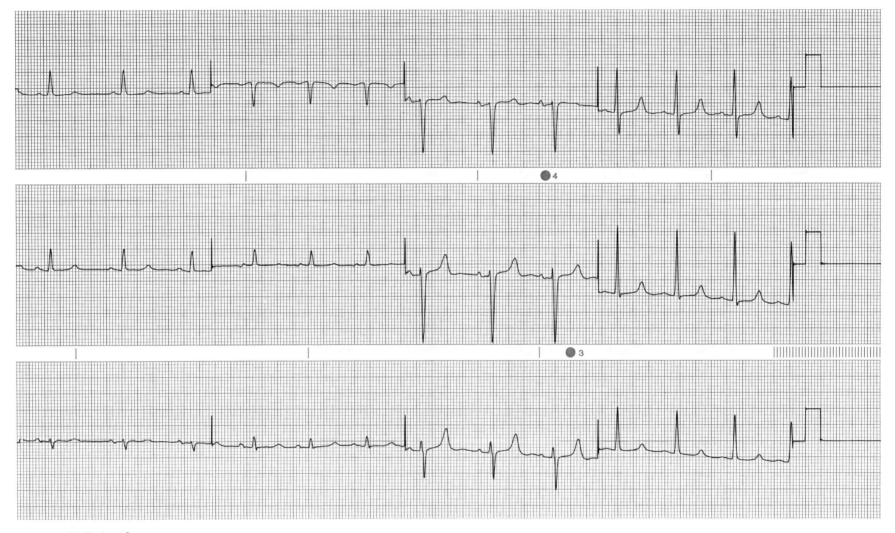

Exercise IX, Patient 9

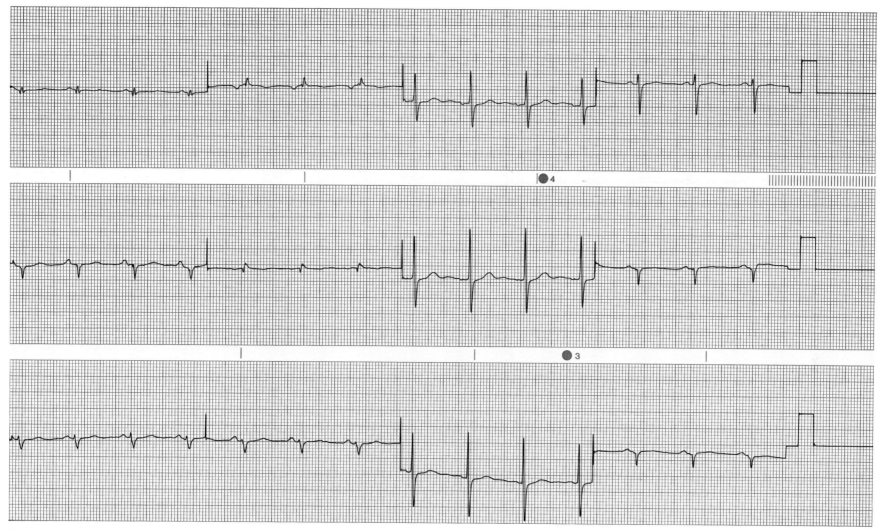

Exercise IX, Patient 10

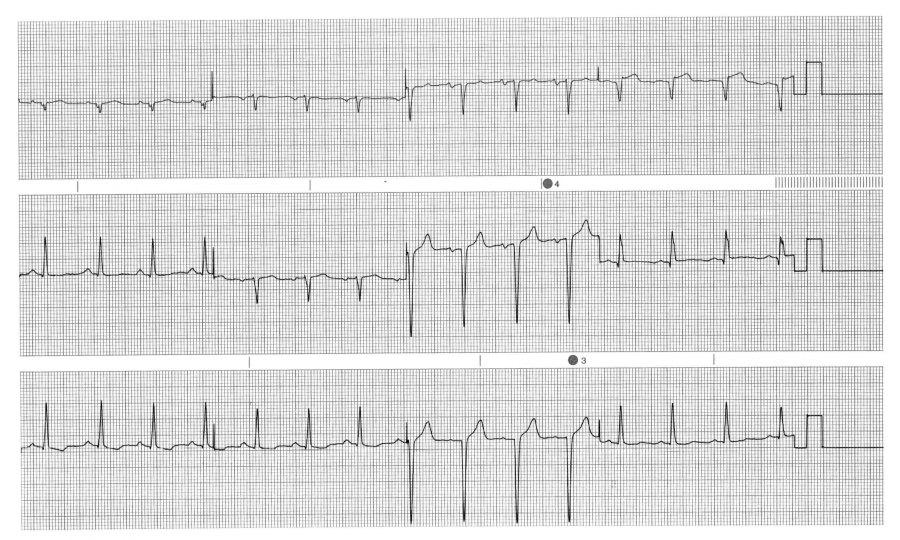

Exercise IX, Patient 11

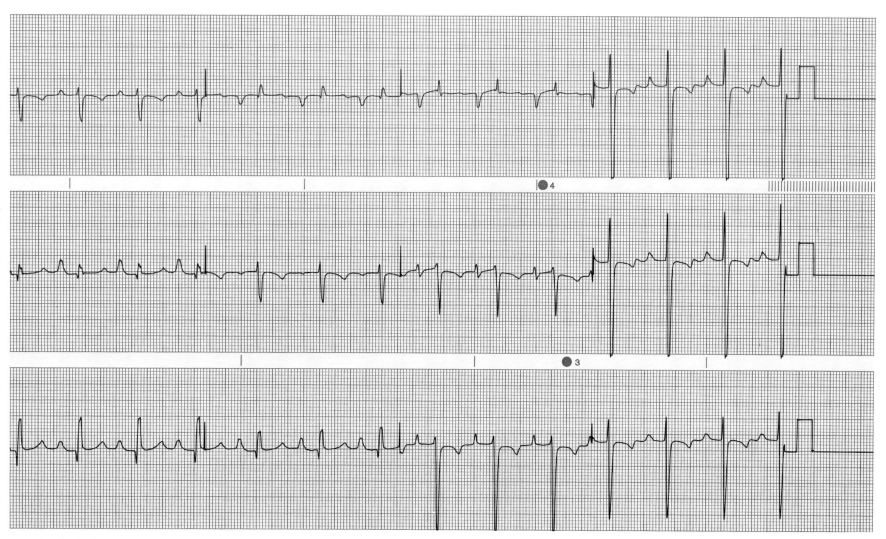

Exercise IX, Patient 12

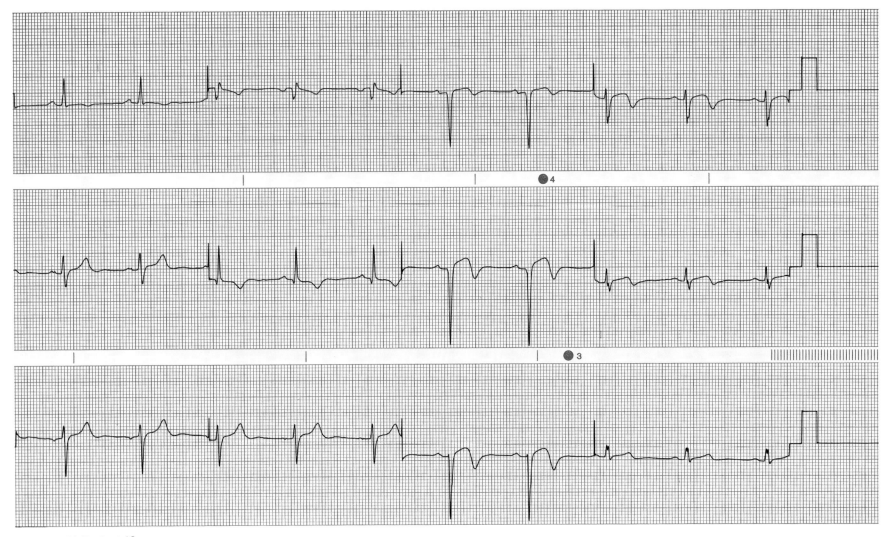

Exercise IX, Patient 13

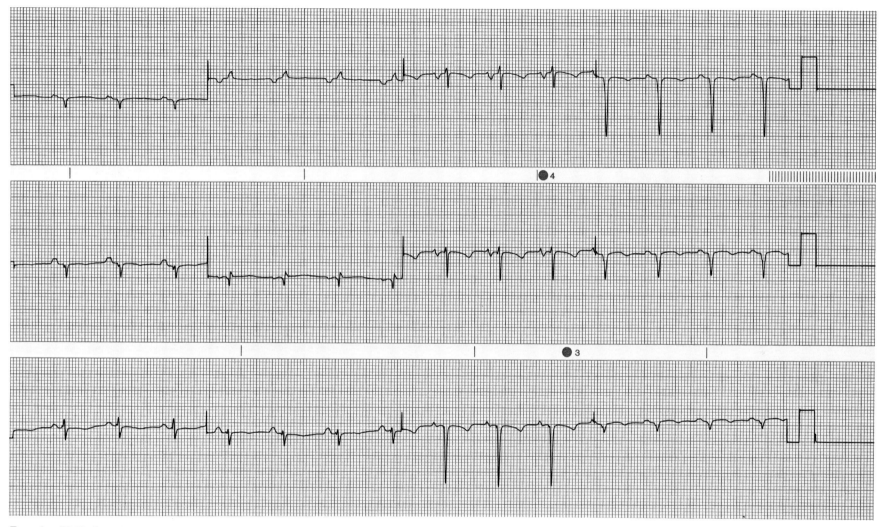

Exercise IX, Patient 14

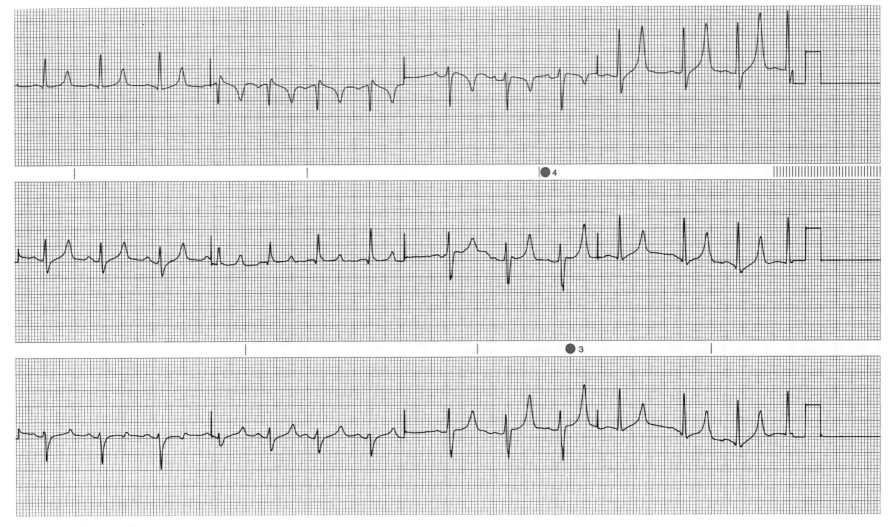

Exercise IX, Patient 15

1. This electrocardiogram shows a sinus rhythm with a first-degree AV block and a right bundle branch block, as evidenced by the widened QRS complex with R′ in lead V_1 and a broad S wave in lead V_6. In addition, there are Q waves in leads II, III, and aV_F and Q waves in leads V_5 and V_6. These are consistent with infarction in the inferior and lateral leads. Coded 6, 41, 55, 77, 78, and 94.

2. This electrocardiogram shows right ventricular hypertrophy with right axis deviation. There is prominent voltage with T wave changes in lead V_1 and especially in lead V_2, and the R wave is less than the S wave in leads V_5 and V_6. Coded 6, 53, 68, and 86.

3. This patient has left atrial enlargement with a prolonged P wave in lead II and a broadly negative P wave in lead V_1. In addition, there is left ventricular hypertrophy diagnosed by the prominent voltage and ST-T wave changes in the lateral leads. Coded 5, 63, 67, and 86.

4. This electrocardiogram suggests a right bundle branch block with lateral infarct but, in fact, is preexcitation. Coded 5 and 47.

5. This is a less specific electrocardiogram. There is poor R wave progression associated with T wave changes and a small Q wave in the aV_L lead. There are nonspecific ST changes in leads V_5 and V_6. This is not inconsistent with a lateral infarction, but is a less firm electrocardiographic diagnosis. Coded 6 and 89 (and probably 77 and 94).

6. This is a wide complex tachycardia. The AV dissociation, which can be seen most clearly in lead II, indicates ventricular tachycardia. The supraventricular rate is rapid and probably represents atrial flutter. Coded 15, 27, and 50.

7. This electrocardiogram shows a sinus rhythm and a complete right bundle branch block. In addition, the ST-T wave changes suggest acute high lateral infarction. There are reciprocal ST segment depressions in leads II, III, and aV_F. Coded 5, 55, 72, 84, and 94.

8. This electrocardiogram shows an anteroseptal myocardial infarction with Q waves in leads V_1 to V_3 and an anterior hemiblock (marked left axis and Q wave in lead aV_L with a QRS duration of <120 milliseconds). Coded 5, 58, 75, and 94.

9. This electrocardiogram shows modest prolongation of the QT interval with symmetric prominence of the T waves. These changes raise the diagnostic possibility of hyperkalemia and hypocalcemia. Coded 5, 91, 92, 97, and 100.

10. This electrocardiogram shows a posterolateral infarction. There are Q waves in leads V_5, V_6, I, and aV_L. There is a Q wave in lead II as well as prominent R forces in leads V_1 and V_2 with upright T waves. This is an example of lead II being associated with lateral infarction. Coded 5, 77, 79, and 94.

11. This patient has an anterolateral infarction with QS waves in leads V_1 to V_4 and I. There is an R wave in lead aV_L. This electrocardiogram does show a right axis and may be an example of posterior hemiblock, although that diagnosis is traditionally made only in the presence of clinical information. Coded 5, 53, 75, and 94 (and possibly 59).

12. This electrocardiogram shows a sinus rhythm with first-degree AV block. There is left atrial enlargement and probably right atrial enlargement from the height of the P wave in lead II and the prominence of P waves in leads V_2 and V_3. Right ventricular hypertrophy is suggested by the prominent R wave in lead V_1, right axis deviation, and a deep S wave in leads V_5 and V_6 associated with T wave changes. Coded 5, 41, 53, 63, and 68 (and possibly 65).

13. This is an anteroseptal myocardial infarction of uncertain age, perhaps recent. There is poor R wave progression, and T waves have terminal, negative symmetry, which extends to lead V_4. In addition, there is left axis, although not enough to diagnose anterior hemiblock. Coded 7, 52, 70, and 94.

14. This electrocardiogram shows an anterolateral infarction with Q waves in leads V_3 through V_6, I, and aV_L. As before, a Q wave in lead II is associated with the lateral infarct. In addition, there is a broad P wave in lead II and a broadly negative P in lead V_1 consistent with left atrial enlargement. Coded 5, 63, 76, 77, and 94.

15. This electrocardiogram shows a sinus rhythm with variation of the RR interval, consistent with sinus arrhythmia. There are prominent symmetric T waves, especially in the lateral leads and relative prolongation of the QT interval. These raise the possibility of hyperkalemia and perhaps also hypocalcemia. Coded 5, 8, 91, 92, and 97 (and possibly 100).

Exercise X

ANSWER SHEET
Exercise X

Patient 1   —— —— —— —— —— —— —— ——

Patient 2   —— —— —— —— —— —— —— ——

Patient 3   —— —— —— —— —— —— —— ——

Patient 4   —— —— —— —— —— —— —— ——

Patient 5   —— —— —— —— —— —— —— ——

Patient 6   —— —— —— —— —— —— —— ——

Patient 7   —— —— —— —— —— —— —— ——

Patient 8   —— —— —— —— —— —— —— ——

Patient 9   —— —— —— —— —— —— —— ——

Patient 10   —— —— —— —— —— —— —— ——

Patient 11   —— —— —— —— —— —— —— ——

Patient 12   —— —— —— —— —— —— —— ——

Patient 13   —— —— —— —— —— —— —— ——

Patient 14   —— —— —— —— —— —— —— ——

Patient 15   —— —— —— —— —— —— —— ——

Electrocardiographic Diagnostic Coding Sheet

General Features
1. Normal ECG
2. Normal ECG, variant
3. Misplaced leads
4. Electrical alternans

Sinus Rhythms
5. Normal sinus
6. Sinus tachycardia
7. Sinus bradycardia
8. Sinus arrhythmia
9. Sinus pause or arrest

Atrial Rhythms
10. Premature atrial contractions (PAC)
11. Aberrant PAC
12. Ectopic atrial rhythm
13. Atrial tachycardia with AV block
14. Atrial fibrillation
15. Atrial flutter
16. Multifocal atrial tachycardia
17. Dual atrial rhythms

AV Junctional Rhythms
18. Premature junctional beats (PJB)
19. Aberrant PJB
20. Junctional beat or rhythm
21. AV junctional rhythm with retrograde atrial activation
22. Supraventricular tachycardia

Ventricular Rhythms
23. Premature ventricular contractions (PVC), unifocal
24. PVC, multifocal
25. PVC, couplets/triplets
26. PVC, R-on-T

27. Ventricular tachycardia
28. Idioventricular rhythm
29. Ventricular fibrillation
30. Ventricular escape beat or rhythm
31. Ventricular fusion beat or rhythm
32. Ventricular capture beat during VT
33. Torsades de pointes

Pacemaker Rhythms
34. Fixed rate
35. Demand
36. Atrial pacing
37. Ventricular pacing
38. Dual chamber pacing
39. Failure to sense
40. Failure to capture

AV Conduction Abnormalities
41. 1° AV block
42. Wenckebach (Mobitz I) AV block
43. 2° AV block (Mobitz II)
44. Fixed 2° AV block, 2:1, 4:1, etc.
45. Complete heart block
46. Variable AV block
47. Preexcitation (WPW)

AV - VA Interactions
48. Fusion beat
49. Echo beat
50. AV dissociation
51. Isorhythmic AV dissociation

Intraventricular Conduction Abnormalities
52. Left axis

53. Right axis
54. Incomplete RBBB
55. Complete RBBB
56. Incomplete LBBB
57. Complete LBBB
58. Anterior hemiblock
59. Posterior hemiblock
60. Nonspecific IVCD
61. Arrhythmia related aberrancy
62. Intermittent IVCD/BBB

Chamber Enlargement
63. Left atrial enlargement
64. Right atrial enlargement
65. Bi-atrial enlargement
66. LVH - voltage
67. LVH - voltage plus repolarization changes
68. RVH
69. Biventricular hypertrophy

Myocardial Infarction

Recent/Acute
70. Anteroseptal
71. Anterior
72. Lateral
73. Inferior
74. Posterior

Old/Uncertain Age
75. Anteroseptal
76. Anterior
77. Lateral
78. Inferior
79. Posterior

Repolarization Changes
80. Possible LV aneurysm
81. Non-Q wave infarction

82. Early repolarization
83. Persistent juvenile T wave
84. ST-T wave changes of acute injury
85. ST-T wave changes of acute ischemia
86. ST-T wave changes of hypertrophy or altered intraventricular conduction (secondary repolarization changes)
87. ST-T wave changes of pericarditis
88. ST changes due to digitalis effect
89. Nonspecific ST-T wave changes
90. Postectopic T wave changes
91. Peaked T waves
92. Prolonged QT interval
93. Prominent U waves

Clinical Problems
94. Coronary artery disease
95. Congenital heart disease
96. Mitral valve disease
97. Hyperkalemia
98. Hypokalemia
99. Hypercalcemia
100. Hypocalcemia
101. Digitalis toxicity
102. CNS event
103. Motion artifact
104. Dextrocardia
105. Cardiac tamponade
106. Cardiac transplant
107. Chronic lung disease

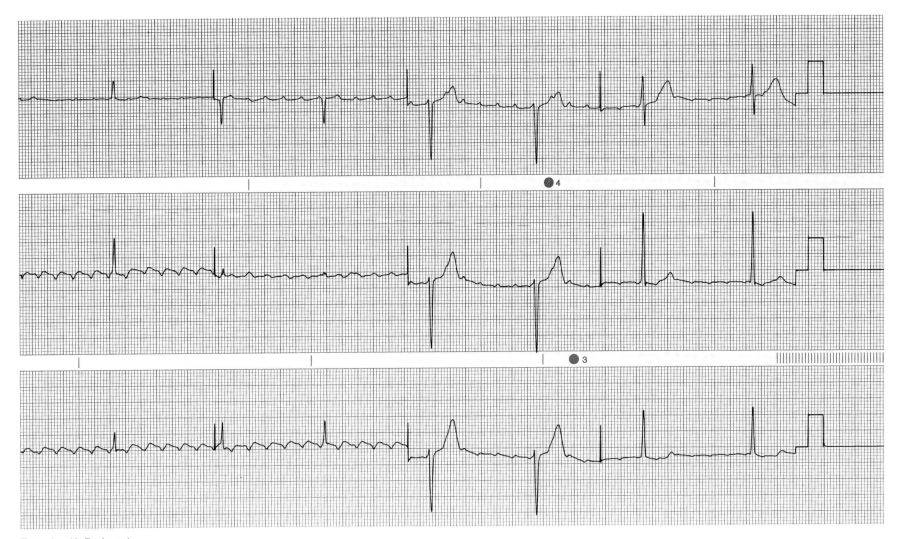

Exercise X, Patient 1

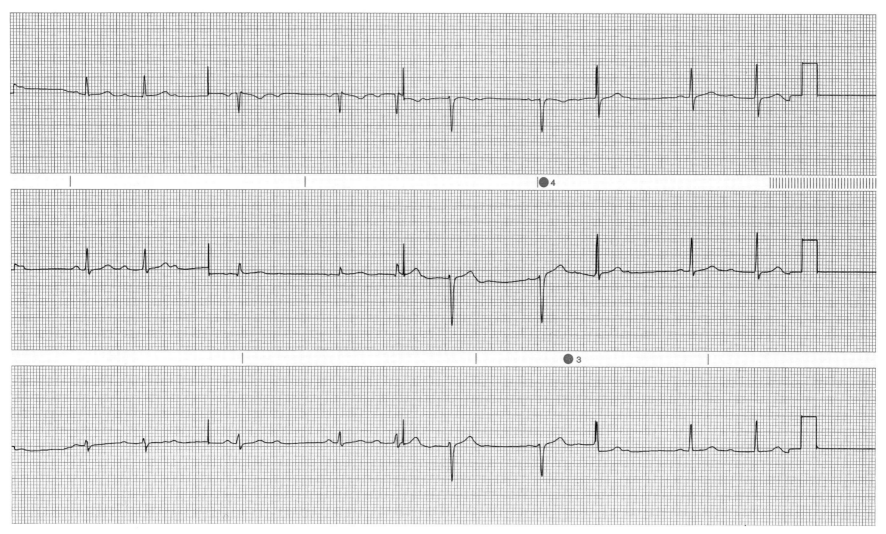

Exercise X, Patient 2

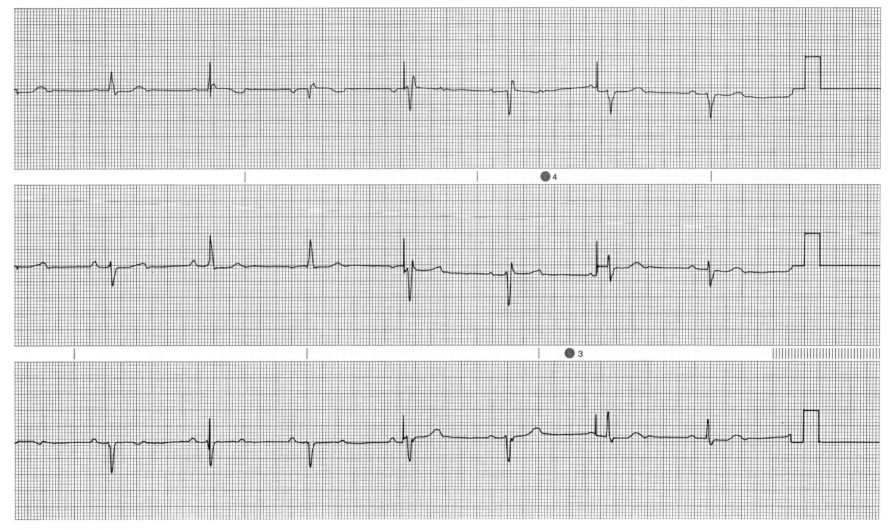

Exercise X, Patient 3

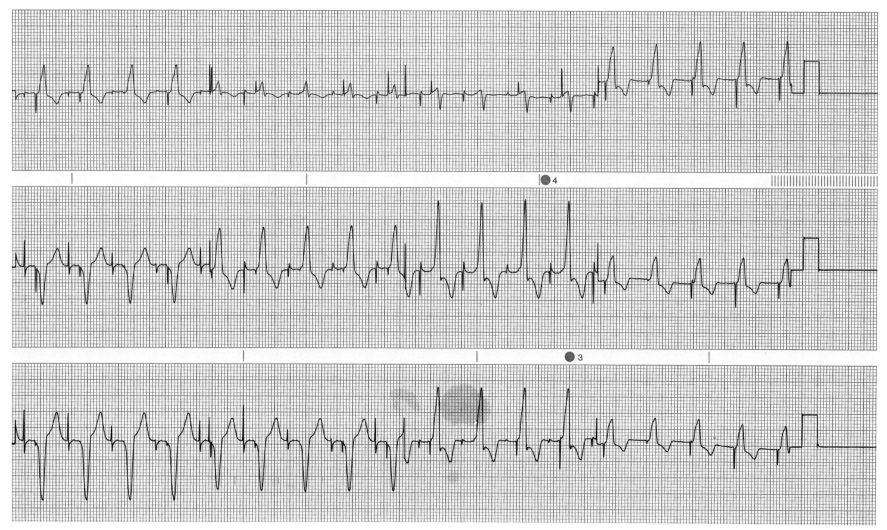

Exercise X, Patient 4

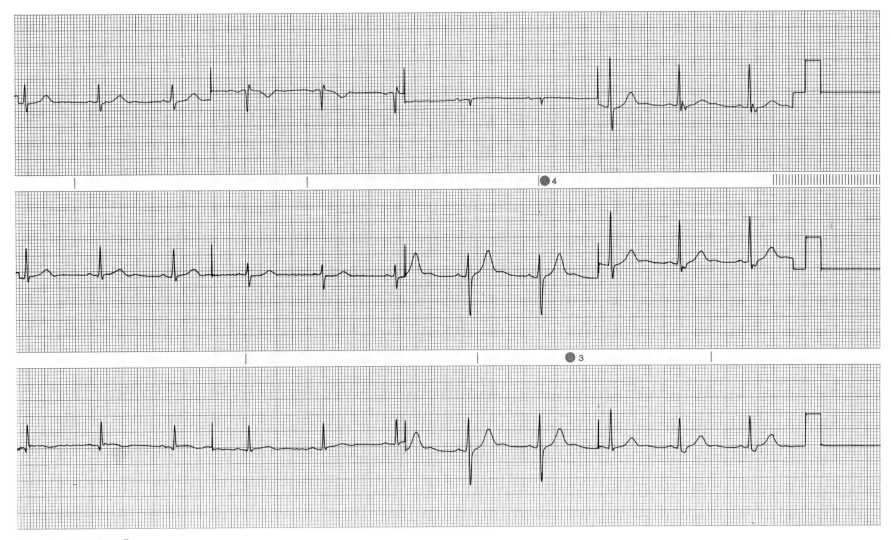

Exercise X, Patient 5

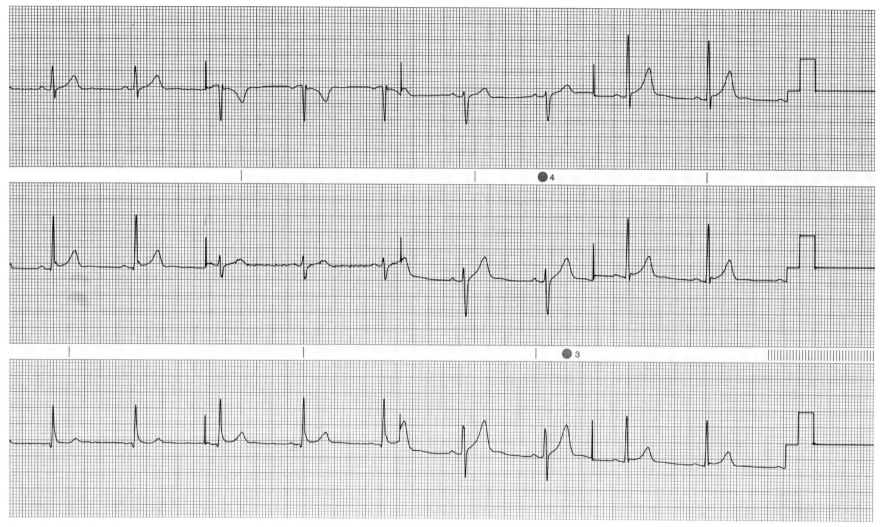

Exercise X, Patient 6

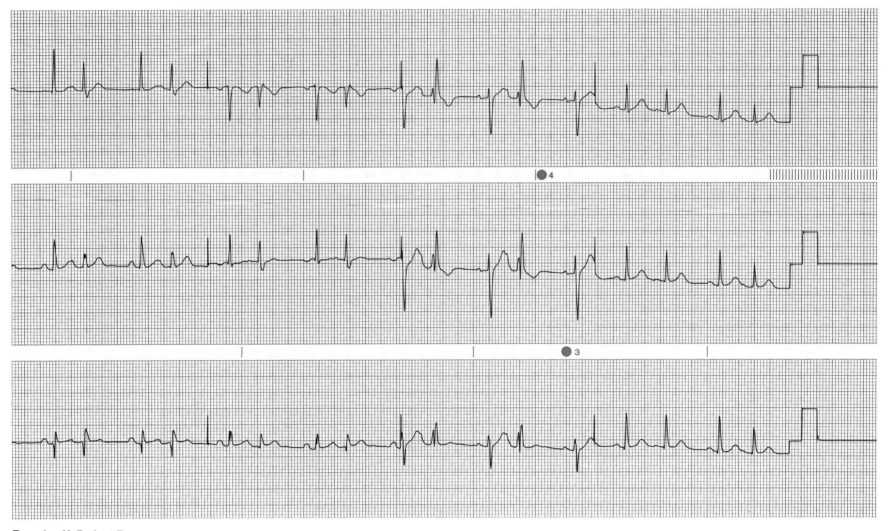

Exercise X, Patient 7

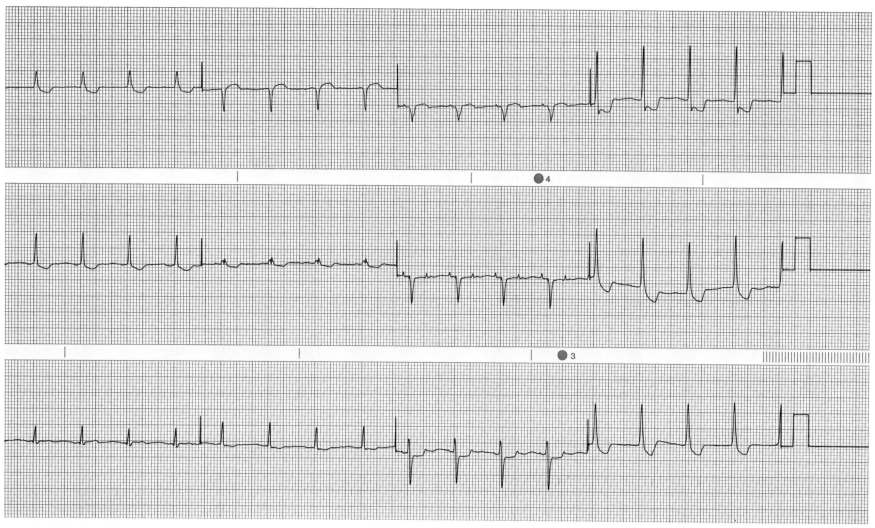

Exercise X, Patient 8

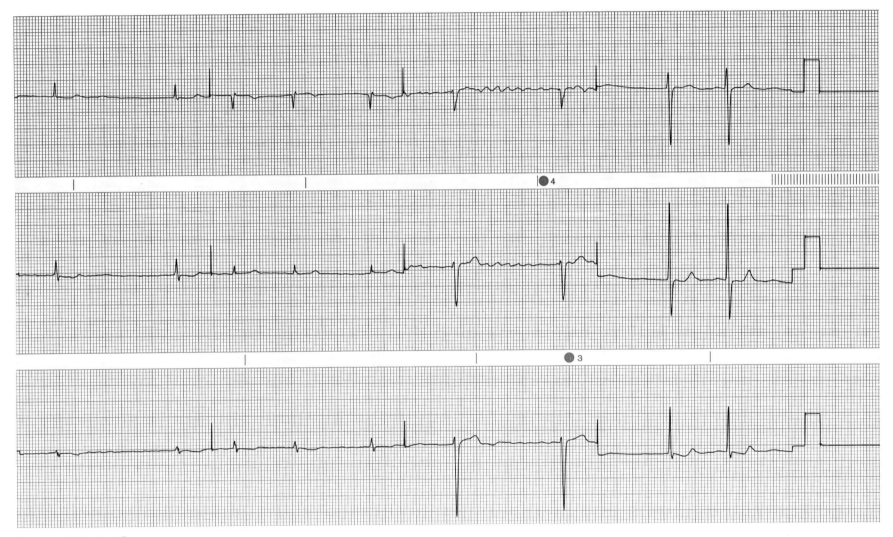

Exercise X, Patient 9

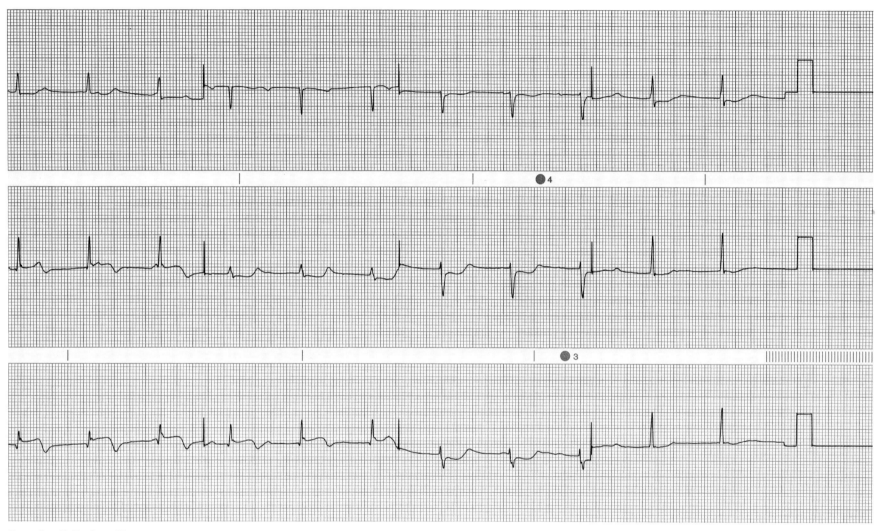

Exercise X, Patient 10

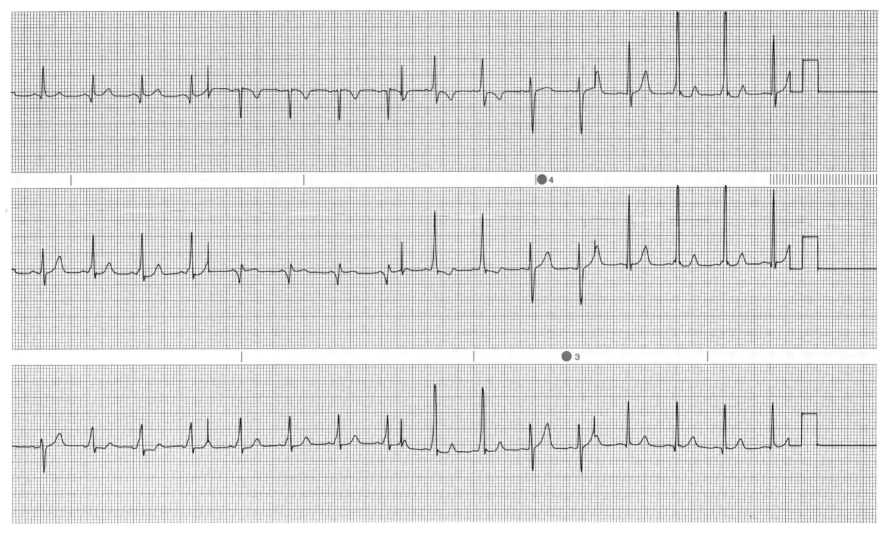

Exercise X, Patient 11

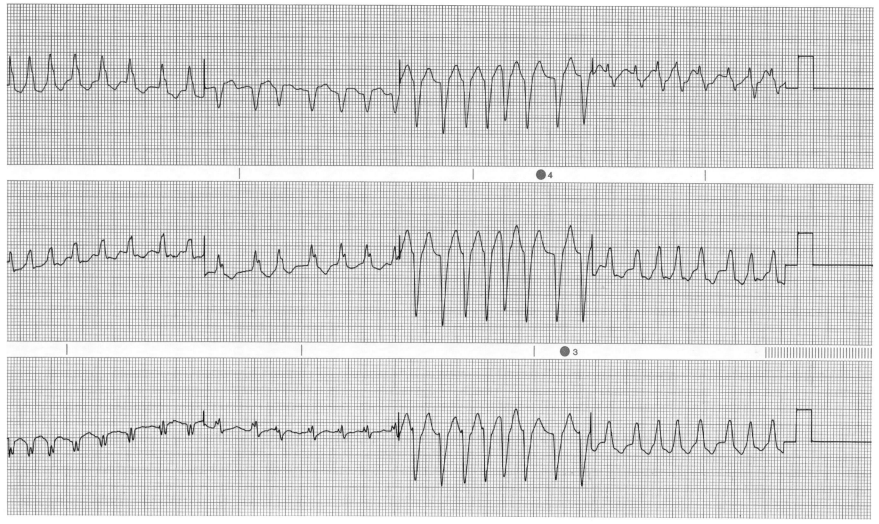

Exercise X, Patient 12

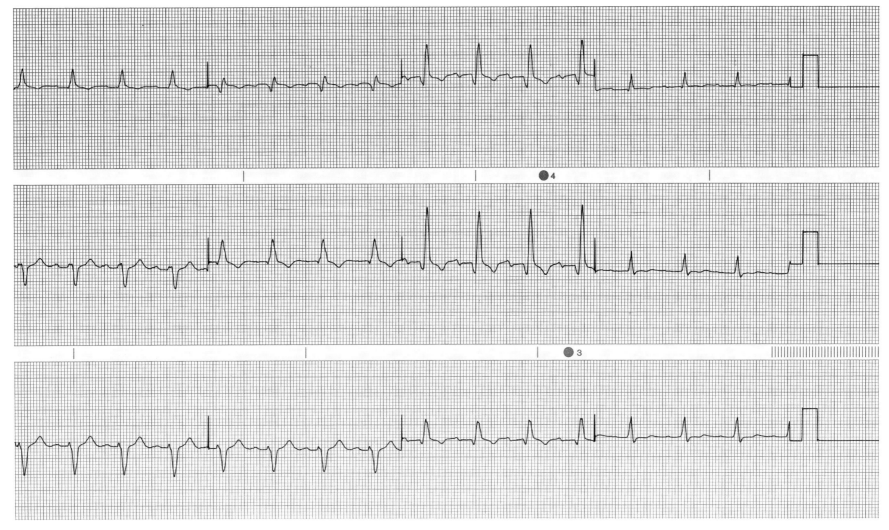

Exercise X, Patient 13

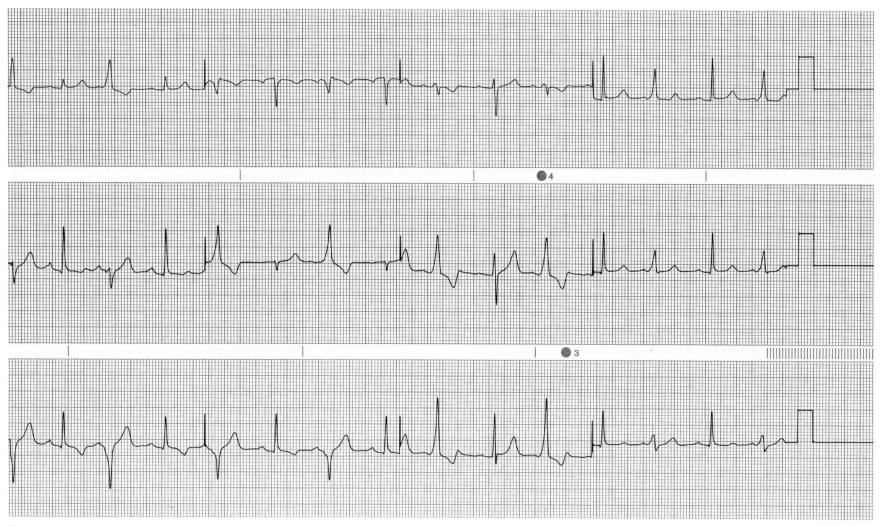

Exercise X, Patient 14

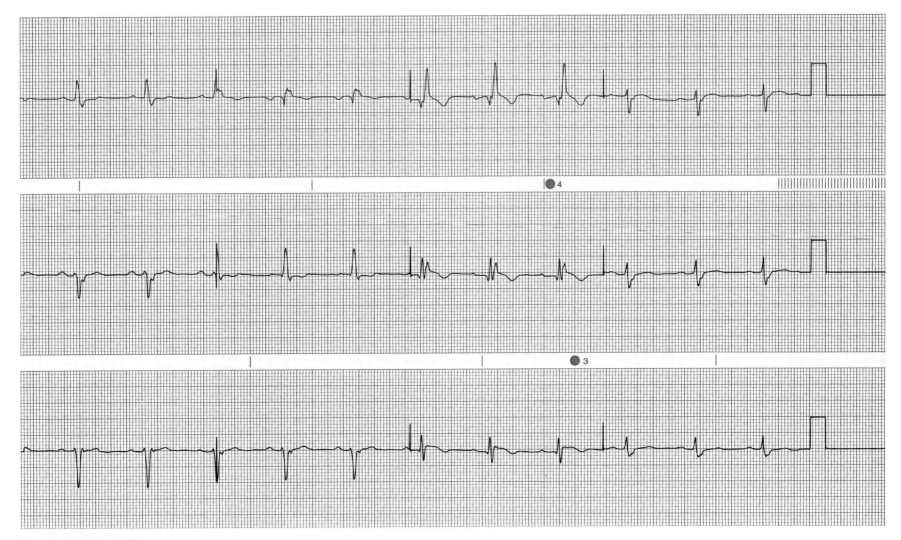

Exercise X, Patient 15

1. This electrocardiogram shows atrial flutter with a variable AV block and nonspecific lateral repolarization abnormalities. Coded 15, 46, and 89.
2. This electrocardiogram shows a sinus rhythm with variable PR intervals and dropped beats, indicating a Wenckebach (Mobitz I) AV block. Coded 5 and 42.
3. This electrocardiogram shows a sinus rhythm with a 2:1 AV block, a right bundle branch block (evident by the R′ in lead V$_1$, broad S wave in lead V$_6$, and the wide QRS complex), and an anterior hemiblock with marked left axis and a small Q wave in lead aV$_L$. R wave regression suggests anterior infarction. In addition, there are nonspecific ST segment changes in the lateral leads. Coded 5, 43, 44, 55, 58, 76, 89, and 94.
4. This is an AV sequential, or at least a dual-chamber, ventricular pacemaker operating 100 percent of the time. Coded 38.
5. This patient has a sinus rhythm and an intermittent complete right bundle branch block, as indicated by the change in width of the QRS complex with a broad terminal S wave in the final two beats of the electrocardiogram. Coded 5, 55, and 62.
6. This electrocardiogram has ST segment elevation in the lateral precordial leads and in leads II and aV$_F$. There are no other abnormalities. The most reasonable diagnosis here is early repolarization, a normal variant. Coded 2, 5, and 82.
7. This normal electrocardiogram has premature atrial beats that are aberrantly and normally conducted. The preceding T wave is distorted by the premature atrial contraction. Coded 1, 5, and 11.
8. This shows atrial tachycardia with AV block. There is ST segment depression with scooping and a short QT interval consistent with digitalis effect. The atrial tachycardia with block raises the possibility of digitalis excess, which was, in fact, the case in this elderly lady with a digoxin level of 4.5 ng/ml. Coded 13, 44, 88, and 101.
9. This electrocardiogram shows atrial fibrillation with a relatively slow ventricular response and ST segment scooping with short QT intervals, suggesting digitalis effect. Coded 14 and 88.
10. This patient has a sinus rhythm with AV dissociation and a nodal escape rhythm. This is due to an acute inferior infarct, suggested by ST segment elevations in leads II, III, and aV$_F$, plus reciprocal ST segment depression in leads aV$_L$, V$_2$, and V$_3$. Coded 5, 20, 50, 73, 84, and 94.
11. This electrocardiogram resembles somewhat right ventricular hypertrophy but instead represents an intermittent Wolff-Parkinson-White syndrome. Characteristic delta waves and short PR intervals are clearly evident in the fourth panel as the second and third of the four beats represented. Coded 5 and 47.
12. This electrocardiogram shows a wide complex tachycardia that is irregularly irregular and has too much RR variability to be ventricular tachycardia. This is actually atrial fibrillation with a left bundle branch block. Coded 14 and 57.
13. This electrocardiogram shows a sinus rhythm with a first-degree AV block. There is a right bundle branch block diagnosed by the wide QRS complex, broad R′ in lead V$_1$, and terminal S in lead V$_6$. There is left axis deviation consistent with left anterior hemiblock as well as Q waves in leads V$_1$ to V$_3$, suggesting anteroseptal myocardial infarction. Coded 5, 41, 55, 58, 75, and 94.
14. This patient has a sinus rhythm and ventricular bigeminy. There are also nonspecific repolarization changes that might be post-ectopic T wave changes, but it is impossible to say in the absence of a series of normally conducted beats. Coded 5, 23, and 89.
15. This electrocardiogram shows sinus rhythm with a right bundle branch block, anterior hemiblock, and anteroseptal myocardial infarction—another bifascicular block caused by coronary disease. Coded 5, 55, 58, 75, and 94.

Exercise XI

ANSWER SHEET
Exercise XI

Patient 1   ___ ___ ___ ___ ___ ___ ___ ___

Patient 2   ___ ___ ___ ___ ___ ___ ___ ___

Patient 3   ___ ___ ___ ___ ___ ___ ___ ___

Patient 4   ___ ___ ___ ___ ___ ___ ___ ___

Patient 5   ___ ___ ___ ___ ___ ___ ___ ___

Patient 6   ___ ___ ___ ___ ___ ___ ___ ___

Patient 7   ___ ___ ___ ___ ___ ___ ___ ___

Patient 8   ___ ___ ___ ___ ___ ___ ___ ___

Patient 9   ___ ___ ___ ___ ___ ___ ___ ___

Patient 10   ___ ___ ___ ___ ___ ___ ___ ___

Patient 11   ___ ___ ___ ___ ___ ___ ___ ___

Patient 12   ___ ___ ___ ___ ___ ___ ___ ___

Patient 13   ___ ___ ___ ___ ___ ___ ___ ___

Patient 14   ___ ___ ___ ___ ___ ___ ___ ___

Patient 15   ___ ___ ___ ___ ___ ___ ___ ___

Electrocardiographic Diagnostic Coding Sheet

General Features
1. Normal ECG
2. Normal ECG, variant
3. Misplaced leads
4. Electrical alternans

Sinus Rhythms
5. Normal sinus
6. Sinus tachycardia
7. Sinus bradycardia
8. Sinus arrhythmia
9. Sinus pause or arrest

Atrial Rhythms
10. Premature atrial contractions (PAC)
11. Aberrant PAC
12. Ectopic atrial rhythm
13. Atrial tachycardia with AV block
14. Atrial fibrillation
15. Atrial flutter
16. Multifocal atrial tachycardia
17. Dual atrial rhythms

AV Junctional Rhythms
18. Premature junctional beats (PJB)
19. Aberrant PJB
20. Junctional beat or rhythm
21. AV junctional rhythm with retrograde atrial activation
22. Supraventricular tachycardia

Ventricular Rhythms
23. Premature ventricular contractions (PVC), unifocal
24. PVC, multifocal
25. PVC, couplets/triplets
26. PVC, R-on-T
27. Ventricular tachycardia
28. Idioventricular rhythm
29. Ventricular fibrillation
30. Ventricular escape beat or rhythm
31. Ventricular fusion beat or rhythm
32. Ventricular capture beat during VT
33. Torsades de pointes

Pacemaker Rhythms
34. Fixed rate
35. Demand
36. Atrial pacing
37. Ventricular pacing
38. Dual chamber pacing
39. Failure to sense
40. Failure to capture

AV Conduction Abnormalities
41. 1° AV block
42. Wenckebach (Mobitz I) AV block
43. 2° AV block (Mobitz II)
44. Fixed 2° AV block, 2:1, 4:1, etc.
45. Complete heart block
46. Variable AV block
47. Preexcitation (WPW)

AV - VA Interactions
48. Fusion beat
49. Echo beat
50. AV dissociation
51. Isorhythmic AV dissociation

Intraventricular Conduction Abnormalities
52. Left axis
53. Right axis
54. Incomplete RBBB
55. Complete RBBB
56. Incomplete LBBB
57. Complete LBBB
58. Anterior hemiblock
59. Posterior hemiblock
60. Nonspecific IVCD
61. Arrhythmia related aberrancy
62. Intermittent IVCD/BBB

Chamber Enlargement
63. Left atrial enlargement
64. Right atrial enlargement
65. Bi-atrial enlargement
66. LVH - voltage
67. LVH - voltage plus repolarization changes
68. RVH
69. Biventricular hypertrophy

Myocardial Infarction
Recent/Acute
70. Anteroseptal
71. Anterior
72. Lateral
73. Inferior
74. Posterior

Old/Uncertain Age
75. Anteroseptal
76. Anterior
77. Lateral
78. Inferior
79. Posterior

Repolarization Changes
80. Possible LV aneurysm
81. Non-Q wave infarction
82. Early repolarization
83. Persistent juvenile T wave
84. ST-T wave changes of acute injury
85. ST-T wave changes of acute ischemia
86. ST-T wave changes of hypertrophy or altered intraventricular conduction (secondary repolarization changes)
87. ST-T wave changes of pericarditis
88. ST changes due to digitalis effect
89. Nonspecific ST-T wave changes
90. Postectopic T wave changes
91. Peaked T waves
92. Prolonged QT interval
93. Prominent U waves

Clinical Problems
94. Coronary artery disease
95. Congenital heart disease
96. Mitral valve disease
97. Hyperkalemia
98. Hypokalemia
99. Hypercalcemia
100. Hypocalcemia
101. Digitalis toxicity
102. CNS event
103. Motion artifact
104. Dextrocardia
105. Cardiac tamponade
106. Cardiac transplant
107. Chronic lung disease

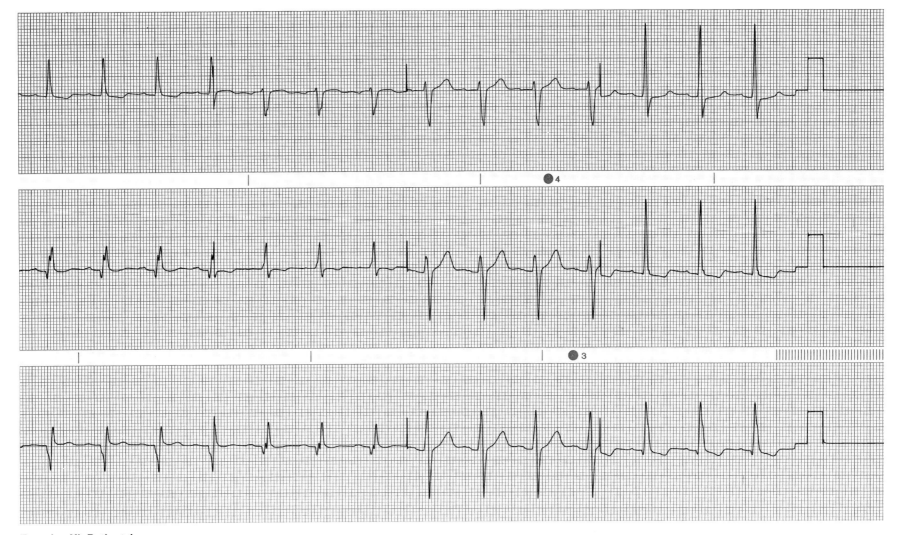

Exercise XI, Patient 1

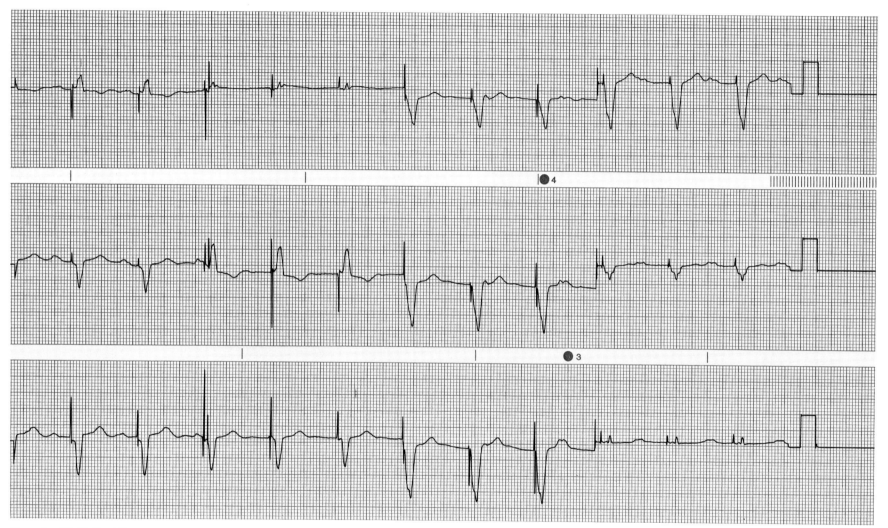

Exercise XI, Patient 2

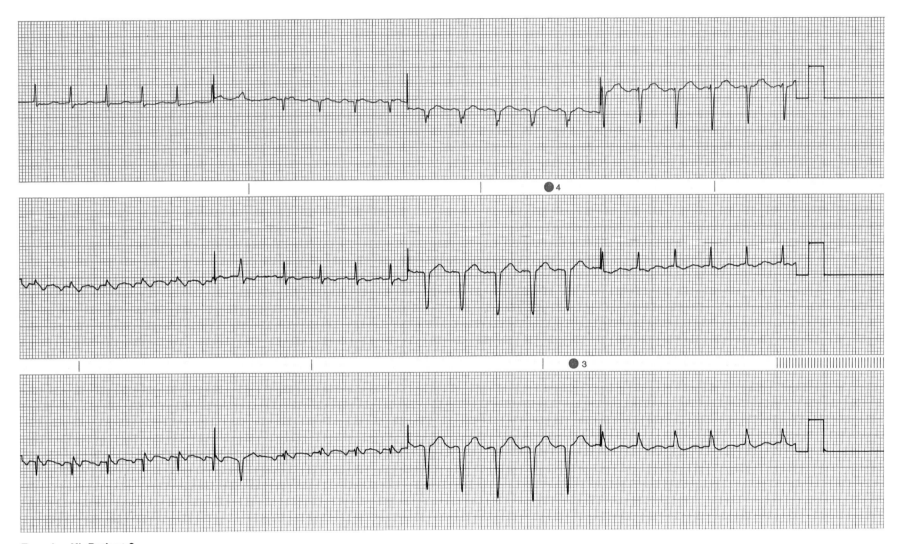

Exercise XI, Patient 3

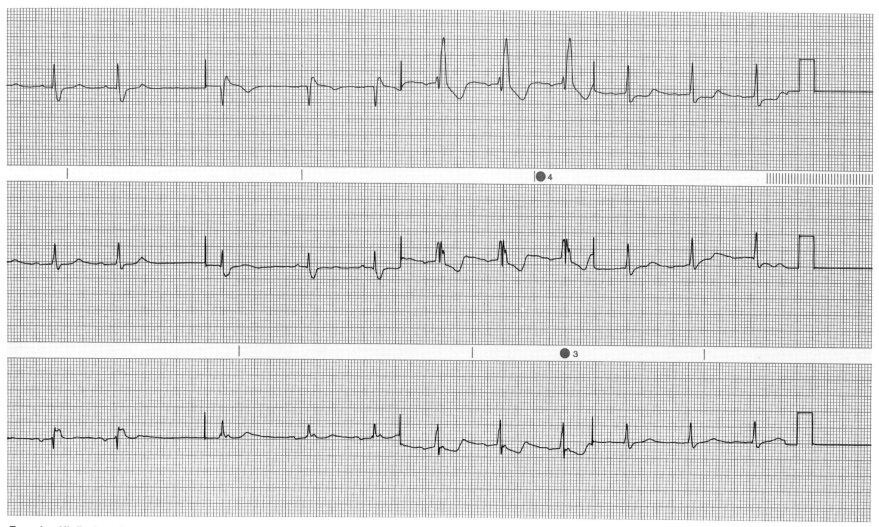

Exercise XI, Patient 4

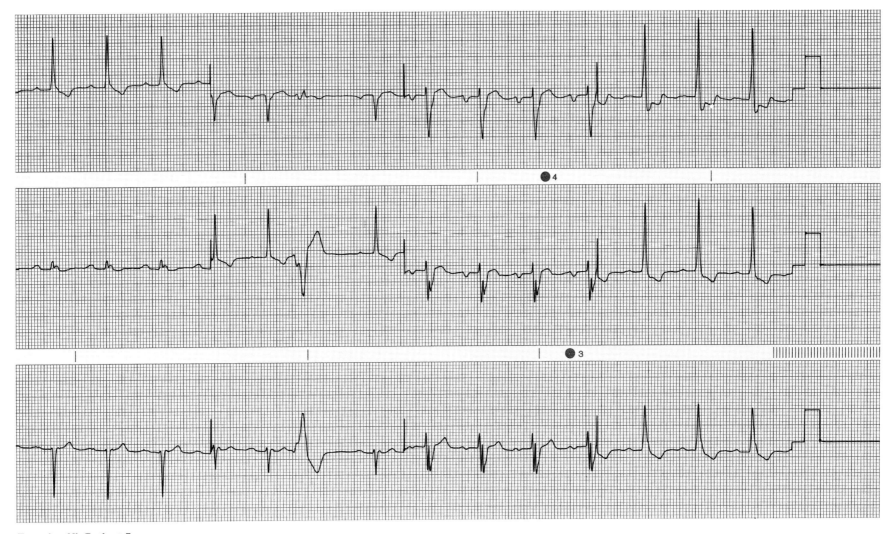

Exercise XI, Patient 5

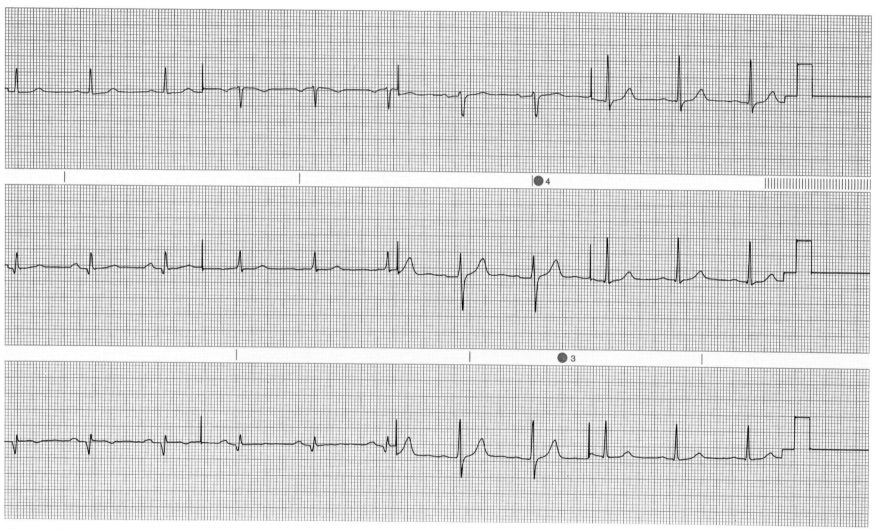

Exercise XI, Patient 6

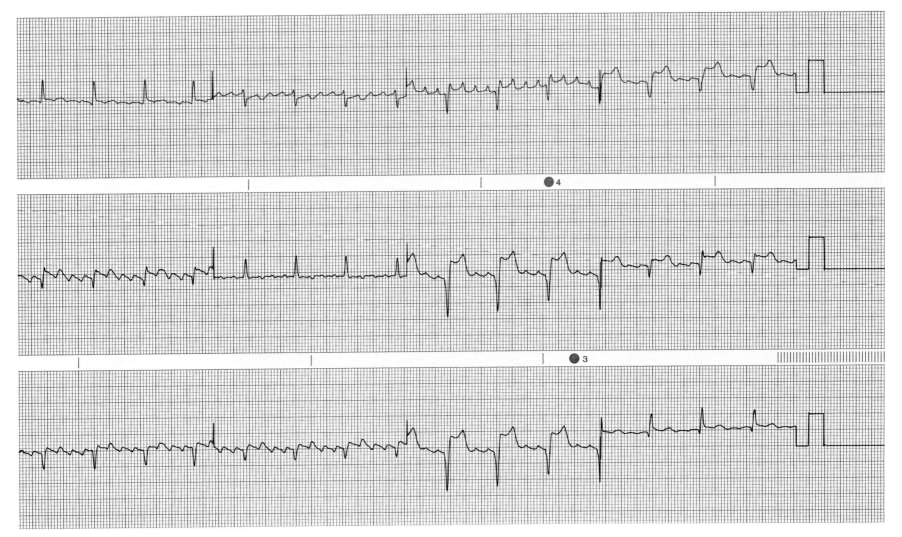

Exercise XI, Patient 7

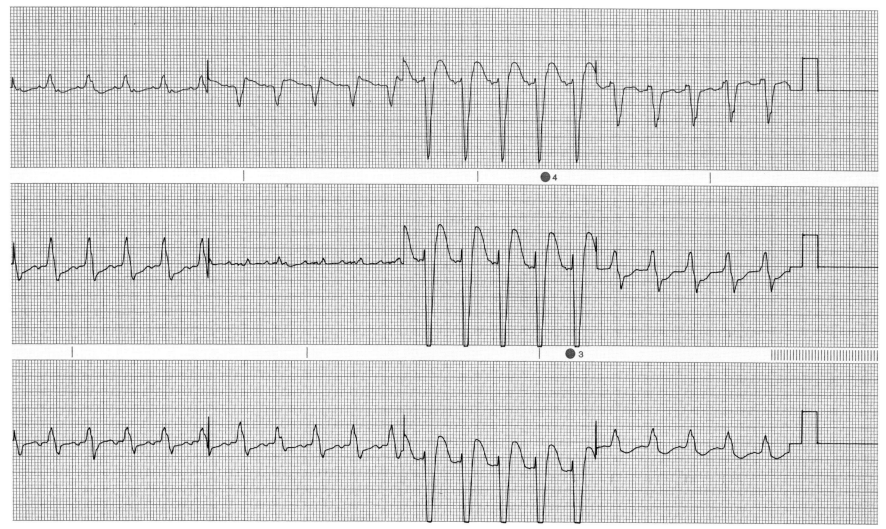

Exercise XI, Patient 8

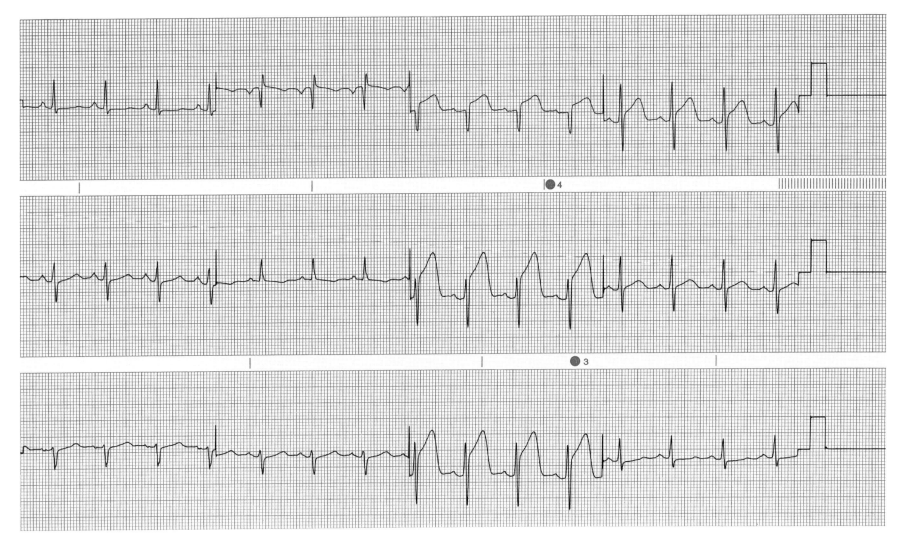

Exercise XI, Patient 9

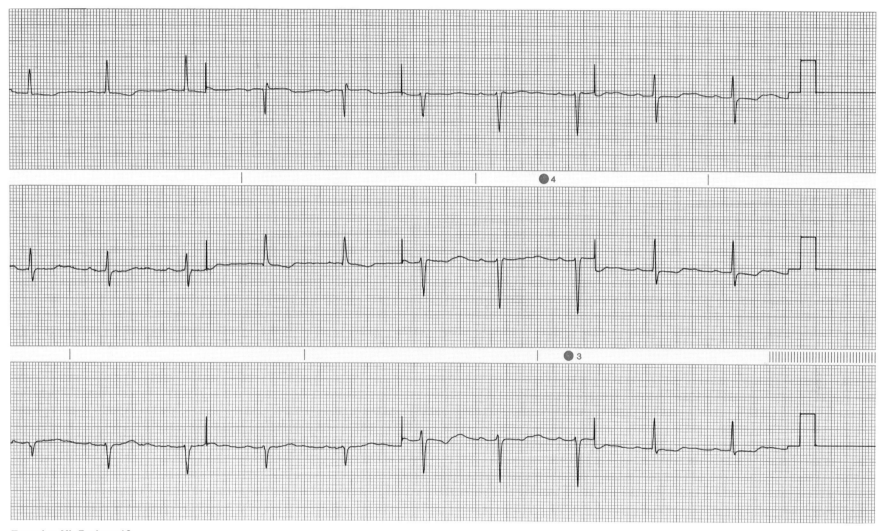

Exercise XI, Patient 10

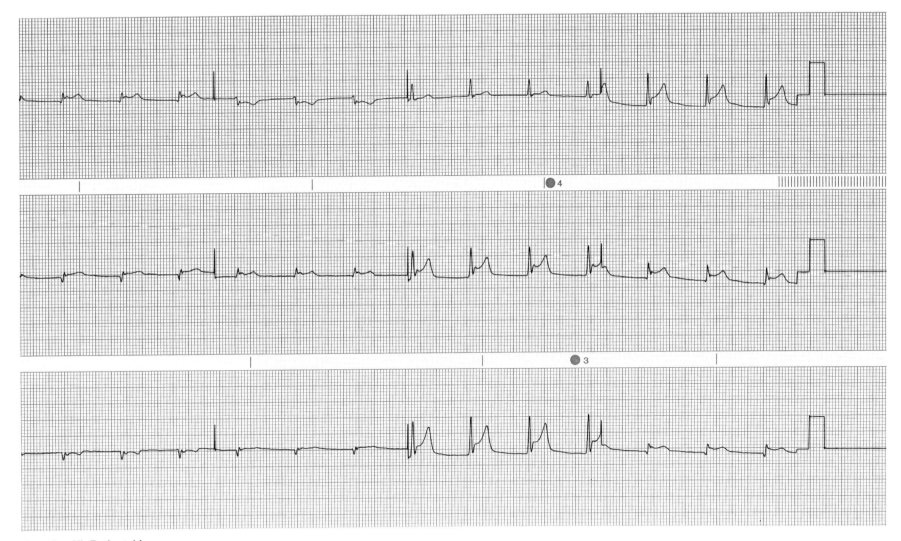

Exercise XI, Patient 11

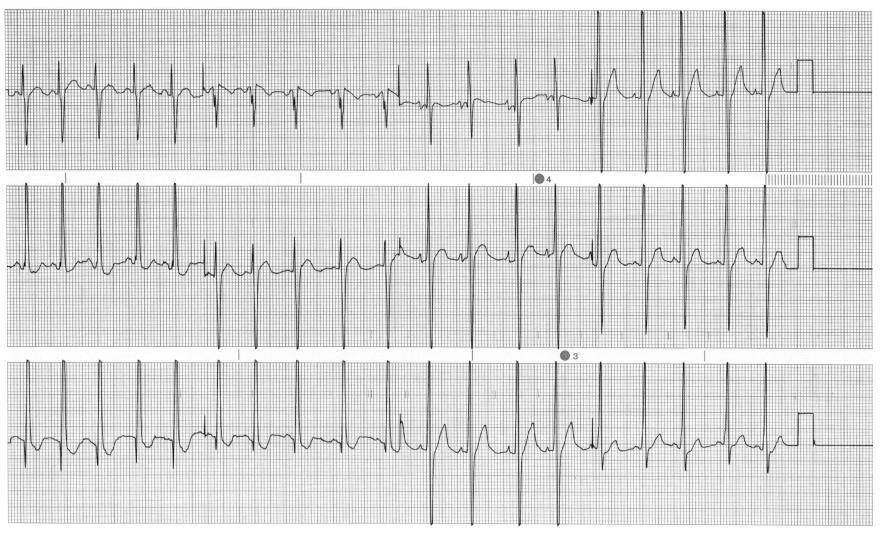

Exercise XI, Patient 12

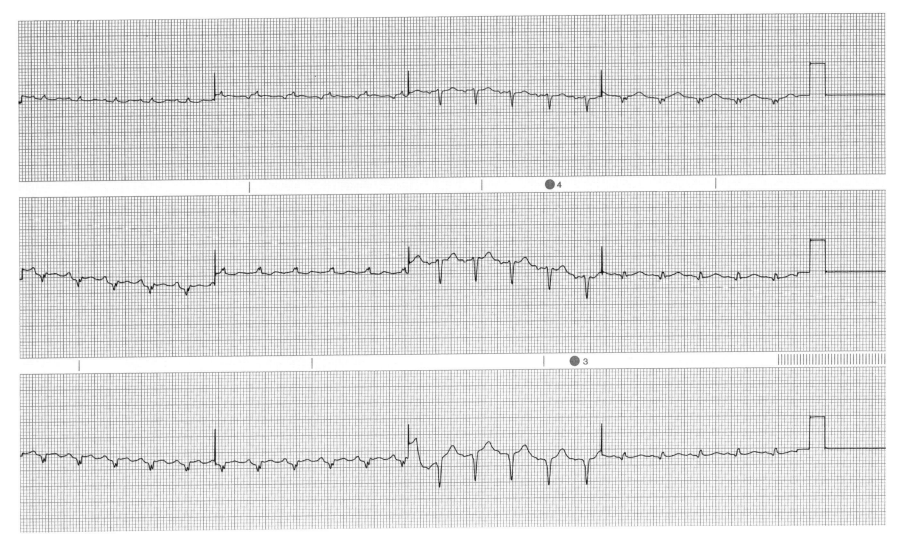

Exercise XI, Patient 13

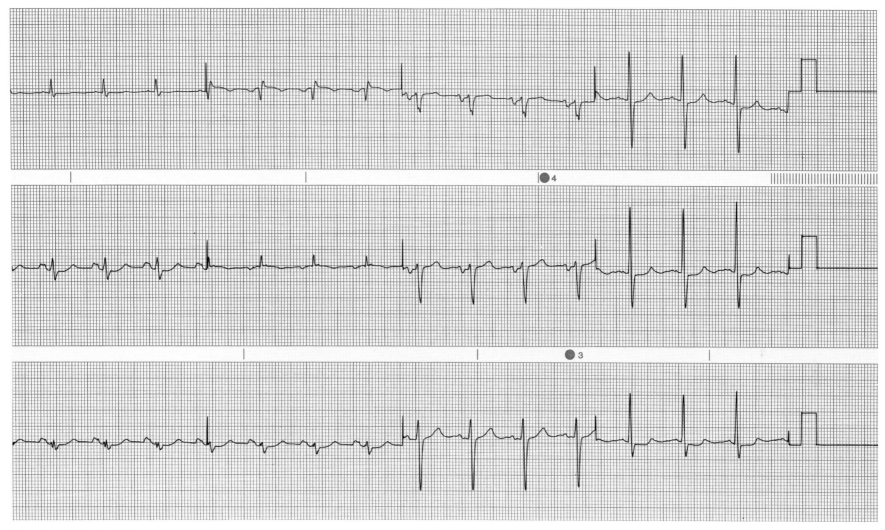

Exercise XI, Patient 14

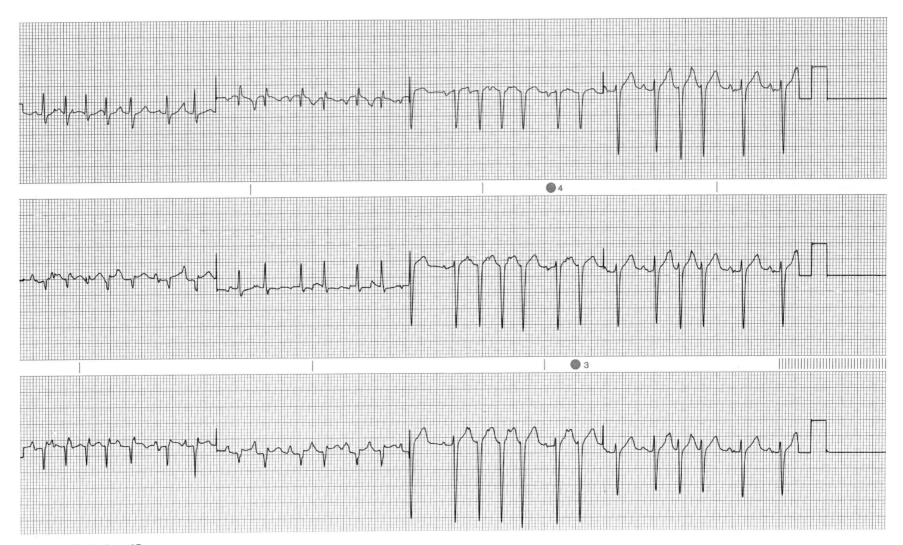

Exercise XI, Patient 15

1. This electrocardiogram shows a sinus rhythm. There are broad Q waves in the inferior leads, consistent with an old inferior myocardial infarction. There is widening of the QRS complex and ST-T wave changes with prominent lateral voltage, all suggesting ventricular hypertrophy. Coded 5, 67, 78, 86, and 94.

2. This is a sinus rhythm with complete heart block and a paced ventricular rhythm. Coded 5, 37, and 45.

3. This electrocardiogram shows atrial flutter with a 2:1 AV block. The flutter waves are best seen in the inferiorly directed leads. In addition, there are Q waves in leads V_1 to V_3, suggesting anteroseptal myocardial infarction. Nonspecific ST-T wave changes are seen laterally. Coded 15, 44, 75, 89, and 94.

4. This patient has a sinus rhythm with a blocked premature atrial contraction following the second beat. This is identified by an altered T wave in that beat compared with the preceding T wave. This is not a sinus pause or arrest. There is right bundle branch block with broad R' in lead V_1, widening of the QRS complex >0.12 second and a wide terminal S wave in lead V_6. There is also a nodal escape beat following the blocked atrial premature contraction (APC). Coded 5, 10, 20, 55, and 86.

5. This patient has a sinus rhythm with a first-degree AV block. P waves are broadly negative in lead V_1, suggesting left atrial enlargement. The QRS complex is widened, and there are T wave and ST segment changes in the lateral leads, which indicate a diagnosis of left ventricular hypertrophy. The absence of Q waves in leads I and V_6, plus the configuration of lead V_6, gives an incomplete left bundle branch block pattern. In addition, there is a premature ventricular beat seen as the third complex in the second panel. Coded 5, 23, 41, 56, 63, 67, and 86.

6. This is a straightforward inferior infarction. The Q wave in lead aV_F is broad, being >0.04 second, and is associated with an abnormal T wave. Coded 5, 78, and 94.

7. This electrocardiogram shows atrial flutter with a 4:1 AV block. There is generalized ST segment elevation consistent with pericarditis. In pericarditis occasionally the aV_L lead is isoelectric, as seen here. There are Q waves in the anterior, lateral, and inferior leads consistent with anterior and inferior infarctions of uncertain age. Coded 15, 44, 76, 78, 87, and 94.

8. This electrocardiogram shows a left bundle branch block. The QRS complex is wide (>120 milliseconds), and there are no Q waves in leads I or V_6. There is atrial tachycardia with a 2:1 block. The P waves are best seen in leads I and aV_L. Coded 13, 44, 57, and 86.

9. This patient has a sinus rhythm and acute anteroseptal infarct with elevations in leads V_1 to V_4, and broad T waves with straightening of the upswing of the T wave. There is left axis present but not enough to code anterior hemiblock. Coded 5, 52, 70, 84, and 94.

10. This patient has sinus bradycardia. There is leftward axis present as well as ST depression with T-U fusion, consistent with hypokalemia. Coded 7, 52, 93, and 98.

11. This patient has a nodal rhythm with an old inferoposterior infarct and pericarditis. Pericarditis is diagnosed by the generalized ST segment elevations. The infarction is of uncertain age. It is established by significant Q waves in lead aV_F and the relatively tall R wave in lead V_1. Coded 20, 78, 79, 87, and 94.

12. This electrocardiogram shows a sinus rhythm with variation in the RR interval, consistent with sinus arrhythmia. There is right axis and prominent voltage in lead V_1 and also in the lateral precordial leads, suggesting biventricular hypertrophy. Coded 6, 8, 53, 69, and 86.

13. This patient's electrocardiogram shows sinus tachycardia, an old inferior infarct, and an old anterior infarct with Q waves in leads V_3 to V_6, II, III, and aV_F. Coded 6, 76, 78, and 94.

14. This electrocardiogram shows a sinus rhythm. There is probable left atrial enlargement since the P wave is broad and somewhat notched in lead II and broadly negative in lead V_1. There are lateral repolarization changes with a scooping quality, possibly from digitalis. Coded 5, 63, and 88.

15. This electrocardiogram is irregularly irregular. Lead V_1 shows at least three foci of atrial activation, suggesting a diagnosis of multifocal atrial tachycardia. There are deep S waves relative to R waves in the lateral leads, which raises the possibility of right ventricular hypertrophy. There are also Q waves in leads II, III, and aV_F, consistent with an inferior infarct. Coded 16, 68, 78, and 94 (and probably 107).

Exercise XII

ANSWER SHEET
Exercise XII

Patient 1   —— —— —— —— —— —— —— ——

Patient 2   —— —— —— —— —— —— —— ——

Patient 3   —— —— —— —— —— —— —— ——

Patient 4   —— —— —— —— —— —— —— ——

Patient 5   —— —— —— —— —— —— —— ——

Patient 6   —— —— —— —— —— —— —— ——

Patient 7   —— —— —— —— —— —— —— ——

Patient 8   —— —— —— —— —— —— —— ——

Patient 9   —— —— —— —— —— —— —— ——

Patient 10   —— —— —— —— —— —— —— ——

Patient 11   —— —— —— —— —— —— —— ——

Patient 12   —— —— —— —— —— —— —— ——

Patient 13   —— —— —— —— —— —— —— ——

Patient 14   —— —— —— —— —— —— —— ——

Patient 15   —— —— —— —— —— —— —— ——

Electrocardiographic Diagnostic Coding Sheet

General Features
1. Normal ECG
2. Normal ECG, variant
3. Misplaced leads
4. Electrical alternans

Sinus Rhythms
5. Normal sinus
6. Sinus tachycardia
7. Sinus bradycardia
8. Sinus arrhythmia
9. Sinus pause or arrest

Atrial Rhythms
10. Premature atrial contractions (PAC)
11. Aberrant PAC
12. Ectopic atrial rhythm
13. Atrial tachycardia with AV block
14. Atrial fibrillation
15. Atrial flutter
16. Multifocal atrial tachycardia
17. Dual atrial rhythms

AV Junctional Rhythms
18. Premature junctional beats (PJB)
19. Aberrant PJB
20. Junctional beat or rhythm
21. AV junctional rhythm with retrograde atrial activation
22. Supraventricular tachycardia

Ventricular Rhythms
23. Premature ventricular contractions (PVC), unifocal
24. PVC, multifocal
25. PVC, couplets/triplets
26. PVC, R-on-T
27. Ventricular tachycardia
28. Idioventricular rhythm
29. Ventricular fibrillation
30. Ventricular escape beat or rhythm
31. Ventricular fusion beat or rhythm
32. Ventricular capture beat during VT
33. Torsades de pointes

Pacemaker Rhythms
34. Fixed rate
35. Demand
36. Atrial pacing
37. Ventricular pacing
38. Dual chamber pacing
39. Failure to sense
40. Failure to capture

AV Conduction Abnormalities
41. 1° AV block
42. Wenckebach (Mobitz I) AV block
43. 2° AV block (Mobitz II)
44. Fixed 2° AV block, 2:1, 4:1, etc.
45. Complete heart block
46. Variable AV block
47. Preexcitation (WPW)

AV - VA Interactions
48. Fusion beat
49. Echo beat
50. AV dissociation
51. Isorhythmic AV dissociation

Intraventricular Conduction Abnormalities
52. Left axis
53. Right axis
54. Incomplete RBBB
55. Complete RBBB
56. Incomplete LBBB
57. Complete LBBB
58. Anterior hemiblock
59. Posterior hemiblock
60. Nonspecific IVCD
61. Arrhythmia related aberrancy
62. Intermittent IVCD/BBB

Chamber Enlargement
63. Left atrial enlargement
64. Right atrial enlargement
65. Bi-atrial enlargement
66. LVH - voltage
67. LVH - voltage plus repolarization changes
68. RVH
69. Biventricular hypertrophy

Myocardial Infarction

Recent/Acute
70. Anteroseptal
71. Anterior
72. Lateral
73. Inferior
74. Posterior

Old/Uncertain Age
75. Anteroseptal
76. Anterior
77. Lateral
78. Inferior
79. Posterior

Repolarization Changes
80. Possible LV aneurysm
81. Non-Q wave infarction
82. Early repolarization
83. Persistent juvenile T wave
84. ST-T wave changes of acute injury
85. ST-T wave changes of acute ischemia
86. ST-T wave changes of hypertrophy or altered intraventricular conduction (secondary repolarization changes)
87. ST-T wave changes of pericarditis
88. ST changes due to digitalis effect
89. Nonspecific ST-T wave changes
90. Postectopic T wave changes
91. Peaked T waves
92. Prolonged QT interval
93. Prominent U waves

Clinical Problems
94. Coronary artery disease
95. Congenital heart disease
96. Mitral valve disease
97. Hyperkalemia
98. Hypokalemia
99. Hypercalcemia
100. Hypocalcemia
101. Digitalis toxicity
102. CNS event
103. Motion artifact
104. Dextrocardia
105. Cardiac tamponade
106. Cardiac transplant
107. Chronic lung disease

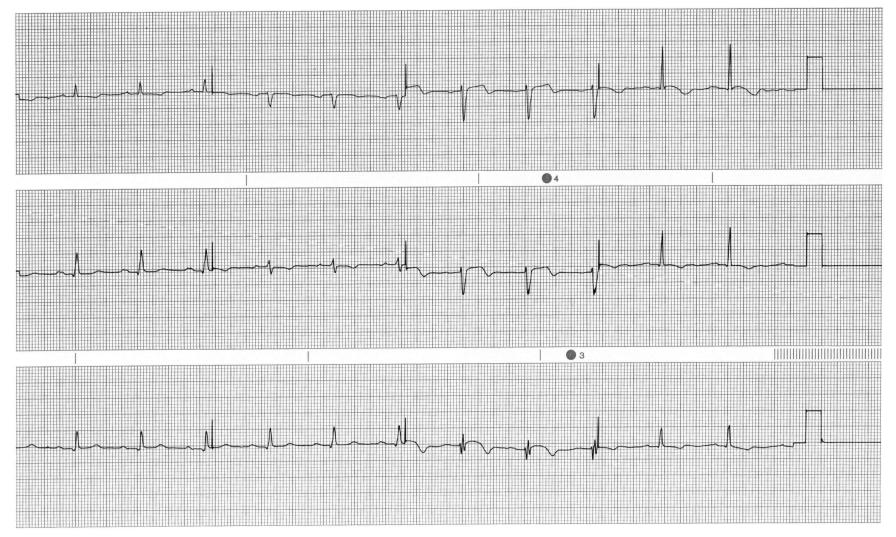

Exercise XII, Patient 1

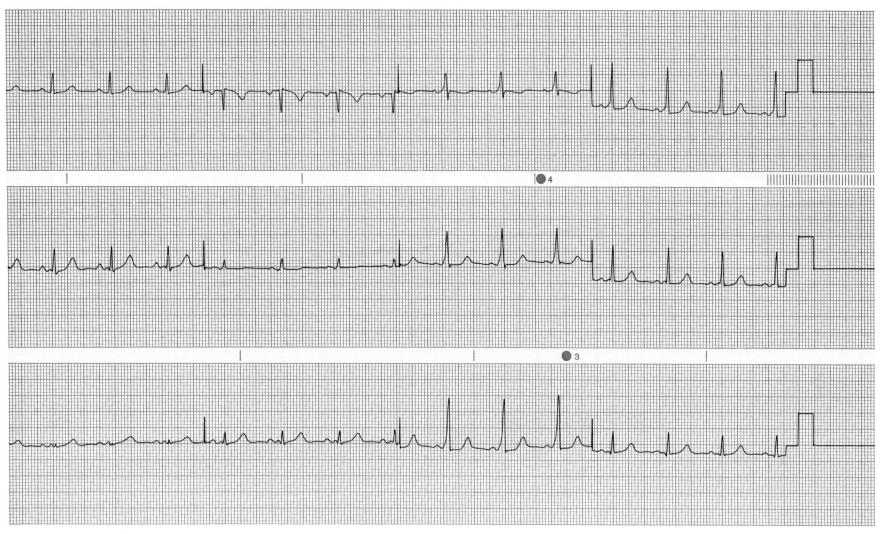

Exercise XII, Patient 2

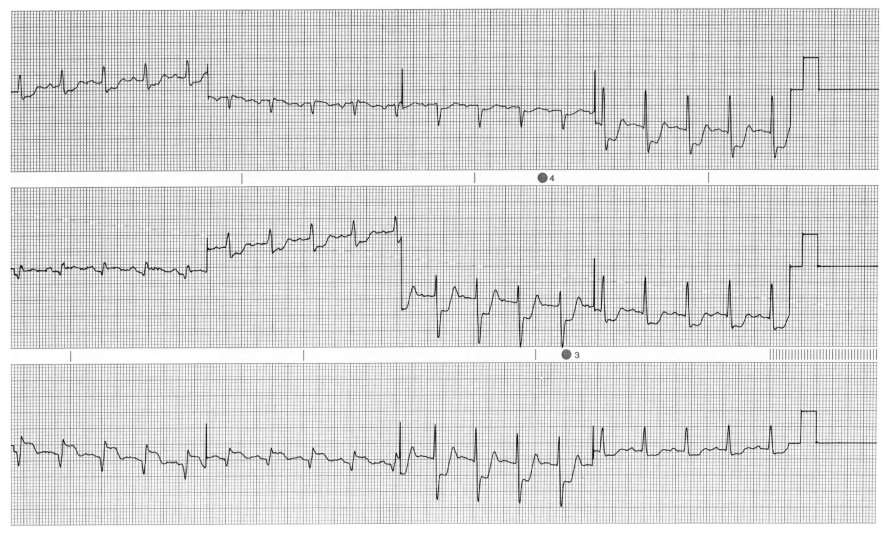

Exercise XII, Patient 3

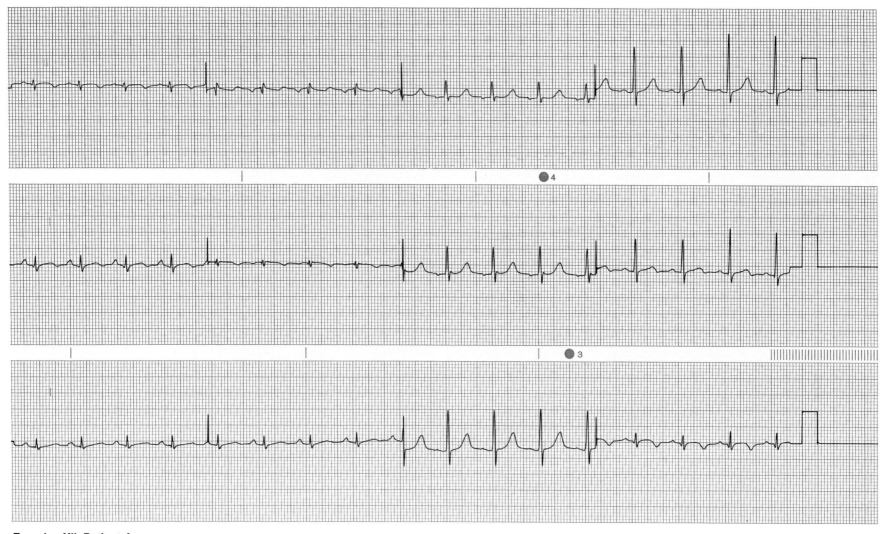

Exercise XII, Patient 4

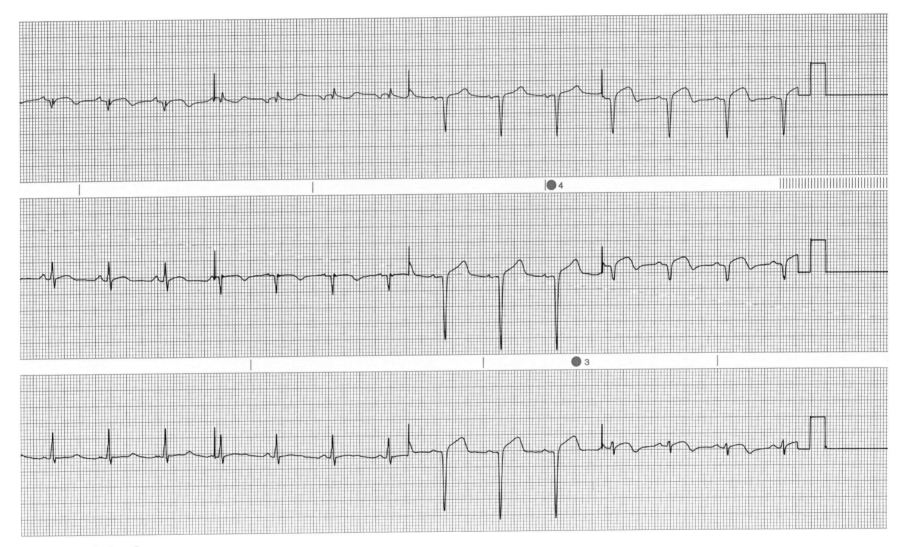

Exercise XII, Patient 5

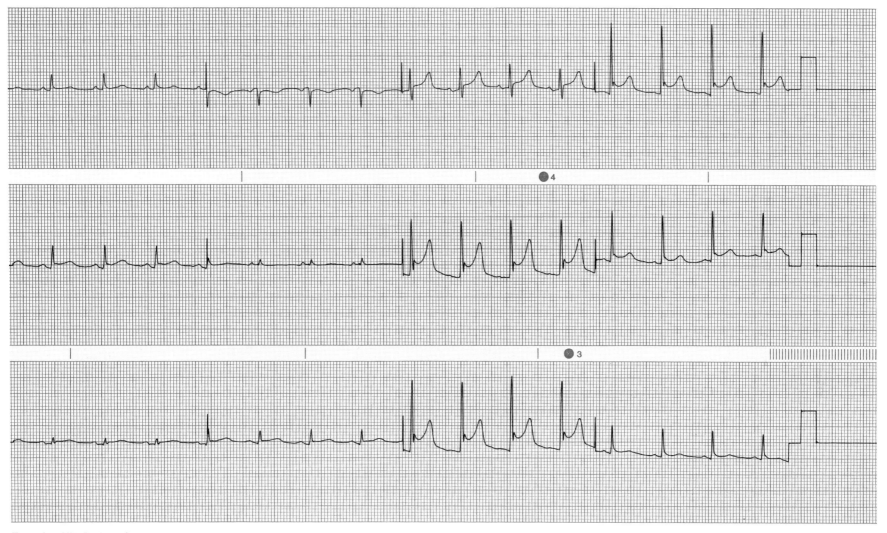

Exercise XII, Patient 6

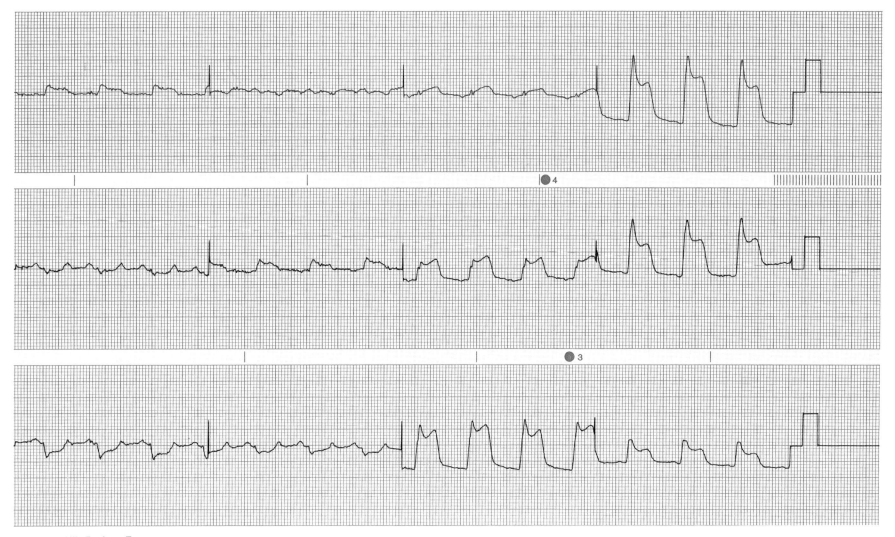

Exercise XII, Patient 7

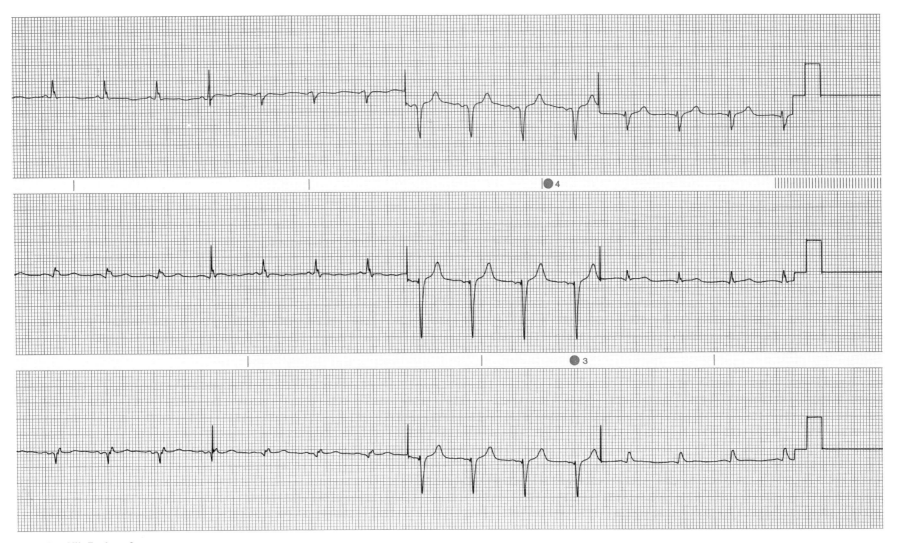

Exercise XII, Patient 8

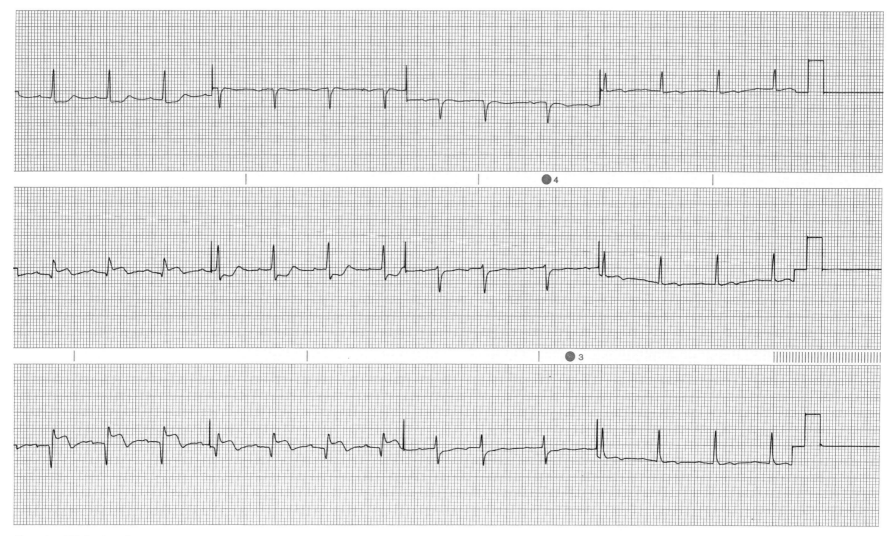

Exercise XII, Patient 9

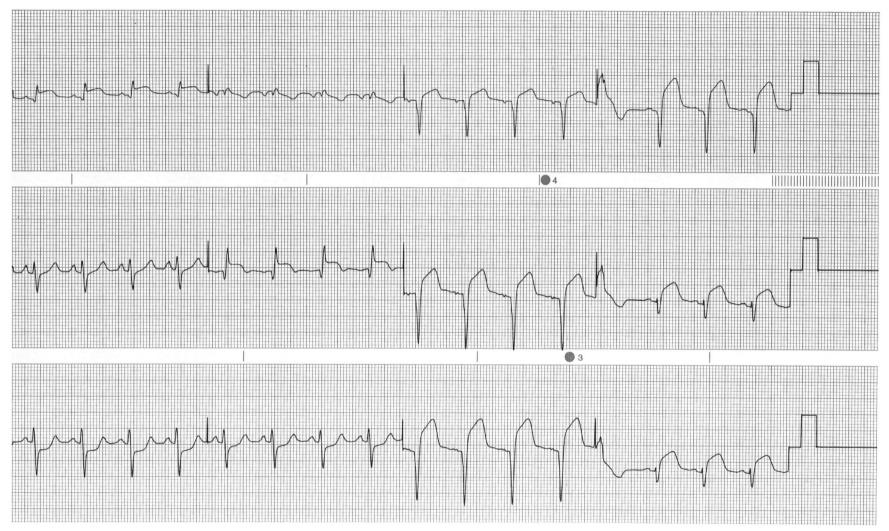

Exercise XII, Patient 10

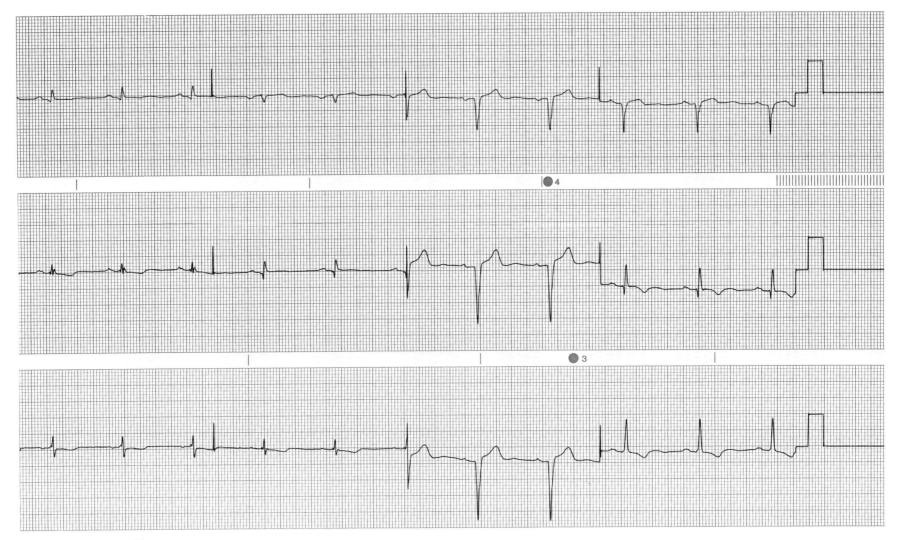

Exercise XII, Patient 11

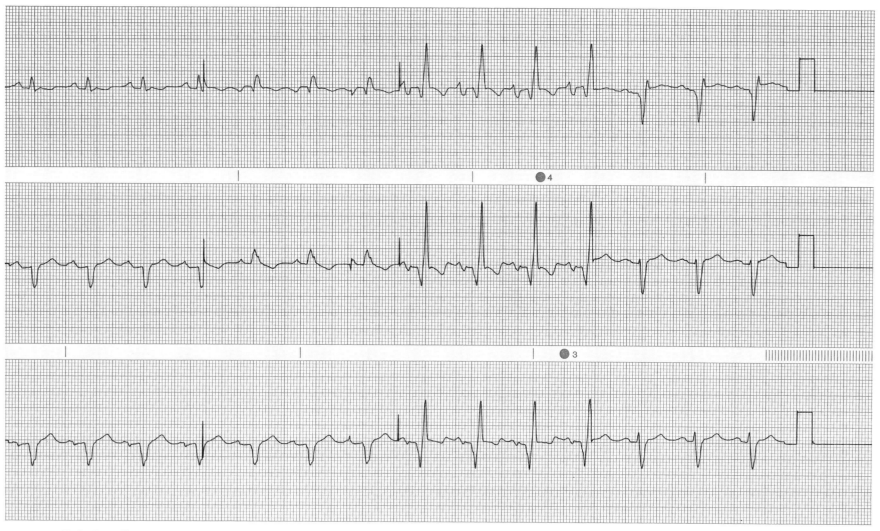

Exercise XII, Patient 12

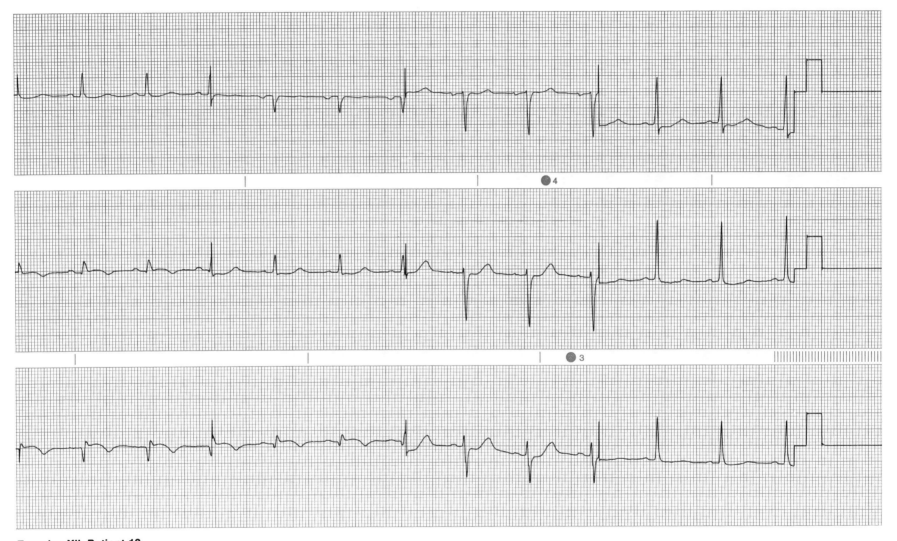

Exercise XII, Patient 13

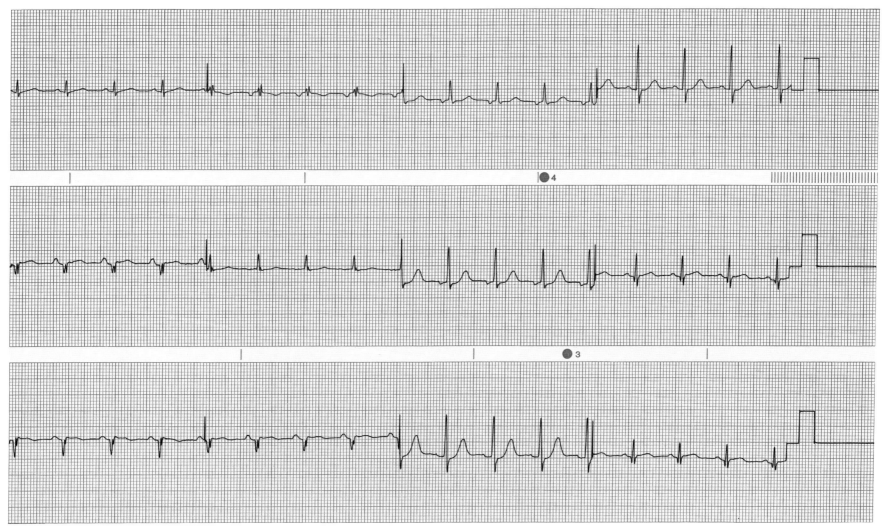

Exercise XII, Patient 14

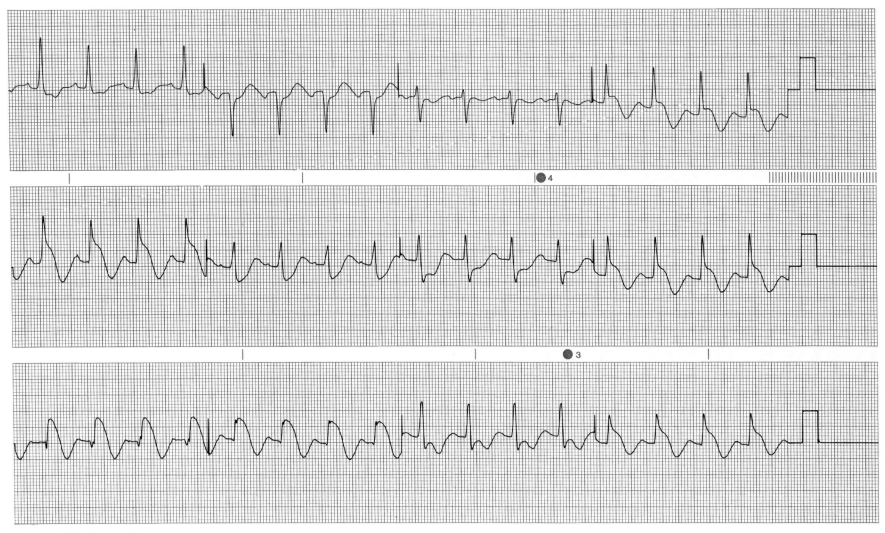

Exercise XII, Patient 15

1. This electrocardiogram shows a sinus rhythm. There is R wave regression with ST segment elevation and T wave inversion in the mid precordial leads. This represents an anterior infarct of uncertain, though probably recent, age. Laterally the ST segment changes are nonspecific. Coded 5, 71, 89, and 94.

2. This electrocardiogram shows Wolff-Parkinson-White syndrome with a pseudo posterior infarct pattern. Delta waves are clearly seen in the right and mid precordial leads. Coded 5 and 47.

3. This electrocardiogram shows an acute inferior infarction. There is sinus tachycardia; marked ST segment elevation in leads III, aV_F, and II; and depressions in leads V_1 to V_6, I, and aV_L. The anterior ST segment depression may represent either reciprocal changes, related to posterior infarct, or to distant ischemia related to associated anterior descending coronary artery disease. Coded 6, 73, 84, and 94.

4. This patient has a sinus rhythm with symmetric T wave inversion in leads V_6 and I. There are prominent anterior forces and counterclockwise rotation. This is a posterolateral infarction of uncertain age, possibly recent in view of the T wave changes in lead V_6. Coded 6, 72, 74, and 94.

5. This is an anterolateral infarction. There are Q waves from leads V_1 to V_5, I, and aV_L and persistent ST segment elevations and T wave changes. This could be a recent event or may represent a left ventricular aneurysm. (Clinically, the age of the infarction would be important in making that diagnosis.) Coded 5, 76, 77, 80, and 94.

6. This is a posterior infarction with pericarditis. There is generalized ST segment elevation, except in leads aV_R and aV_L. The R waves are prominent in lead V_1, and T waves are upright, consistent with posterior myocardial infarction. Coded 5, 79, 87, and 94.

7. This electrocardiogram shows an acute anterior infarction. It has marked ST segment elevation in the precordial and lateral leads and reciprocal depression in the inferior leads. The rhythm is sinus. Coded 5, 71, 72, 84, and 94.

8. This shows old anteroseptal and old inferior infarctions. There are broad Q waves in lead aV_F, supporting a diagnosis of inferior infarct. There are qrS patterns in leads V_2, V_3, and V_4, which in a male are diagnostic with high specificity for anteroseptal infarction. Coded 5, 75, 78, and 94.

9. This electrocardiogram shows an acute inferior infarction. The rhythm is sinus with first-degree AV block. There is a premature atrial contraction as the second beat in the third panel. There is ST segment elevation with evolving T wave changes in leads II, III, and aV_F, and reciprocal depression in leads I and aV_L. Coded 5, 10, 41, 73, 84, and 94.

10. This is an acute anterolateral infarction with a premature ventricular contraction (PVC) and an anterior hemiblock. The rhythm is sinus. The PVC is the first beat in the fourth panel. There is left axis deviation with a Q wave in lead aV_L and a QRS duration of <120 milliseconds. Anteriorly, ST segment elevation is seen in leads I and aV_L. Coded 5, 23, 58, 71, 72, 84, and 94.

11. This is an old anteroseptal infarction with Q waves in leads V_1 to V_4. There are nonspecific repolarization changes laterally. Coded 5, 75, 89, and 94.

12. This electrocardiogram shows a right bundle branch block with inferior and anteroseptal infarctions. There is also left atrial enlargement. Right bundle branch block is diagnosed by the wide complex (>120 milliseconds), the broad R' in lead V_1, and the broad terminal S wave in lead V_6. Left atrial enlargement is based on the very wide negative terminal component of the P wave in lead V_1. There are Q waves in leads V_1 to V_4 and in leads II, III, and aV_F. Coded 5, 55, 63, 75, 78, and 94.

13. This electrocardiogram shows a sinus rhythm, an acute inferior infarction, and nonspecific repolarization changes laterally. The Q waves are developing in the inferior leads with persistent ST segment elevation and symmetric terminal T wave inversion in leads II, III, and aV_F. Coded 5, 73, 84, 89, and 94.

14. This electrocardiogram shows a sinus rhythm and an old inferoposterior infarction. The R wave in lead V_1 is tall, and the T wave upright. There are broad Q waves in inferior leads II, III, and aV_F. Coded 5, 78, 79, and 94.

15. This electrocardiogram shows sinus rhythm with acute inferior and lateral infarctions. There is ST segment elevation in the inferior and lateral leads. The QT interval is prolonged. Reciprocal changes are seen in leads I and V_2. Coded 5, 72, 73, 84, 92, and 94.

Exercise XIII

ANSWER SHEET
Exercise XIII

Patient 1 —— —— —— —— —— —— —— ——

Patient 2 —— —— —— —— —— —— —— ——

Patient 3 —— —— —— —— —— —— —— ——

Patient 4 —— —— —— —— —— —— —— ——

Patient 5 —— —— —— —— —— —— —— ——

Patient 6 —— —— —— —— —— —— —— ——

Patient 7 —— —— —— —— —— —— —— ——

Patient 8 —— —— —— —— —— —— —— ——

Patient 9 —— —— —— —— —— —— —— ——

Patient 10 —— —— —— —— —— —— —— ——

Patient 11 —— —— —— —— —— —— —— ——

Patient 12 —— —— —— —— —— —— —— ——

Patient 13 —— —— —— —— —— —— —— ——

Patient 14 —— —— —— —— —— —— —— ——

Patient 15 —— —— —— —— —— —— —— ——

Electrocardiographic Diagnostic Coding Sheet

General Features
1. Normal ECG
2. Normal ECG, variant
3. Misplaced leads
4. Electrical alternans

Sinus Rhythms
5. Normal sinus
6. Sinus tachycardia
7. Sinus bradycardia
8. Sinus arrhythmia
9. Sinus pause or arrest

Atrial Rhythms
10. Premature atrial contractions (PAC)
11. Aberrant PAC
12. Ectopic atrial rhythm
13. Atrial tachycardia with AV block
14. Atrial fibrillation
15. Atrial flutter
16. Multifocal atrial tachycardia
17. Dual atrial rhythms

AV Junctional Rhythms
18. Premature junctional beats (PJB)
19. Aberrant PJB
20. Junctional beat or rhythm
21. AV junctional rhythm with retrograde atrial activation
22. Supraventricular tachycardia

Ventricular Rhythms
23. Premature ventricular contractions (PVC), unifocal
24. PVC, multifocal
25. PVC, couplets/triplets
26. PVC, R-on-T
27. Ventricular tachycardia
28. Idioventricular rhythm
29. Ventricular fibrillation
30. Ventricular escape beat or rhythm
31. Ventricular fusion beat or rhythm
32. Ventricular capture beat during VT
33. Torsades de pointes

Pacemaker Rhythms
34. Fixed rate
35. Demand
36. Atrial pacing
37. Ventricular pacing
38. Dual chamber pacing
39. Failure to sense
40. Failure to capture

AV Conduction Abnormalities
41. 1° AV block
42. Wenckebach (Mobitz I) AV block
43. 2° AV block (Mobitz II)
44. Fixed 2° AV block, 2:1, 4:1, etc.
45. Complete heart block
46. Variable AV block
47. Preexcitation (WPW)

AV - VA Interactions
48. Fusion beat
49. Echo beat
50. AV dissociation
51. Isorhythmic AV dissociation

Intraventricular Conduction Abnormalities
52. Left axis
53. Right axis
54. Incomplete RBBB
55. Complete RBBB
56. Incomplete LBBB
57. Complete LBBB
58. Anterior hemiblock
59. Posterior hemiblock
60. Nonspecific IVCD
61. Arrhythmia related aberrancy
62. Intermittent IVCD/BBB

Chamber Enlargement
63. Left atrial enlargement
64. Right atrial enlargement
65. Bi-atrial enlargement
66. LVH - voltage
67. LVH - voltage plus repolarization changes
68. RVH
69. Biventricular hypertrophy

Myocardial Infarction
Recent/Acute
70. Anteroseptal
71. Anterior
72. Lateral
73. Inferior
74. Posterior

Old/Uncertain Age
75. Anteroseptal
76. Anterior
77. Lateral
78. Inferior
79. Posterior

Repolarization Changes
80. Possible LV aneurysm
81. Non-Q wave infarction
82. Early repolarization
83. Persistent juvenile T wave
84. ST-T wave changes of acute injury
85. ST-T wave changes of acute ischemia
86. ST-T wave changes of hypertrophy or altered intraventricular conduction (secondary repolarization changes)
87. ST-T wave changes of pericarditis
88. ST changes due to digitalis effect
89. Nonspecific ST-T wave changes
90. Postectopic T wave changes
91. Peaked T waves
92. Prolonged QT interval
93. Prominent U waves

Clinical Problems
94. Coronary artery disease
95. Congenital heart disease
96. Mitral valve disease
97. Hyperkalemia
98. Hypokalemia
99. Hypercalcemia
100. Hypocalcemia
101. Digitalis toxicity
102. CNS event
103. Motion artifact
104. Dextrocardia
105. Cardiac tamponade
106. Cardiac transplant
107. Chronic lung disease

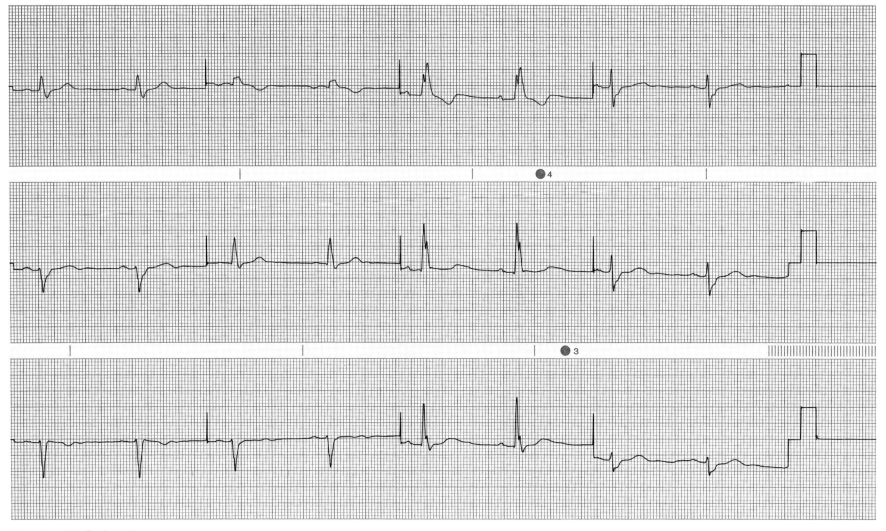

Exercise XIII, Patient 1

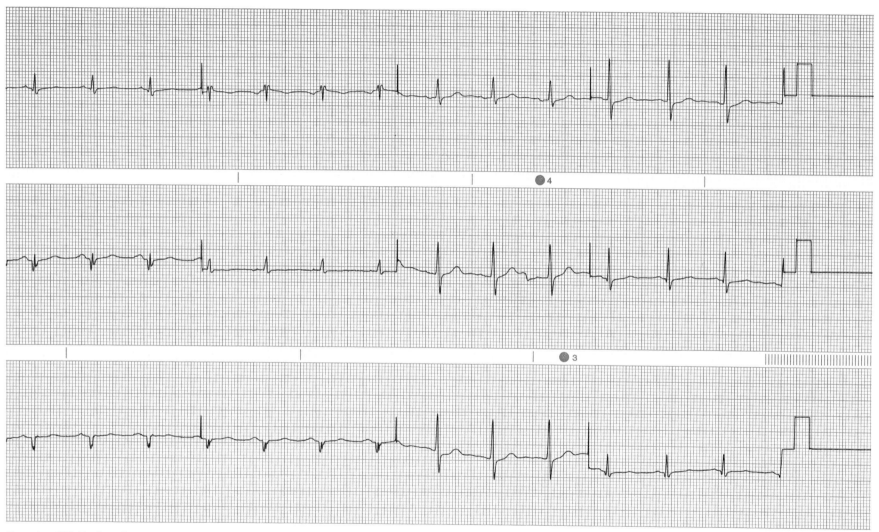

Exercise XIII, Patient 2

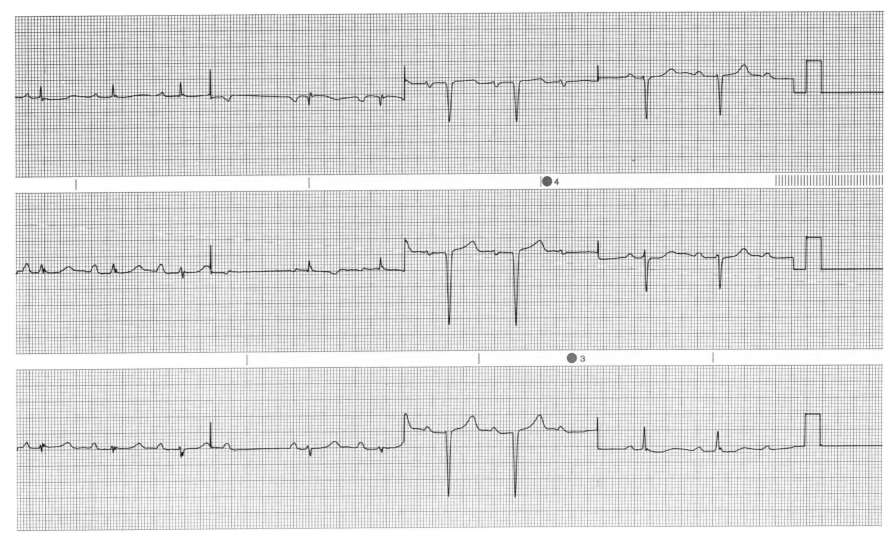

Exercise XIII, Patient 3

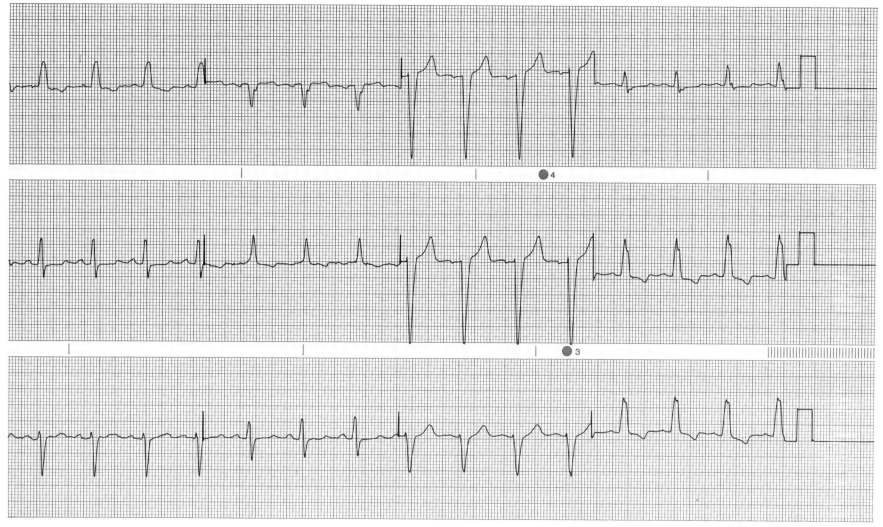

Exercise XIII, Patient 4

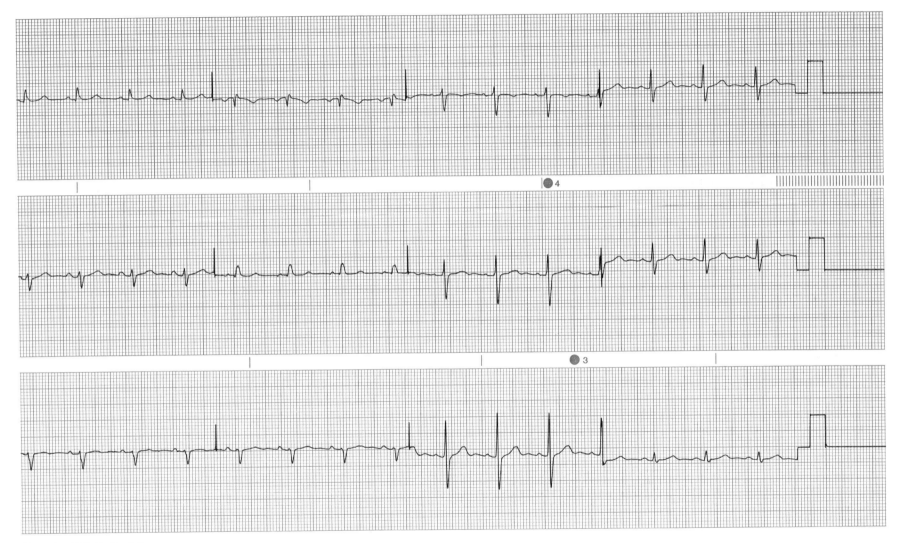

Exercise XIII, Patient 5

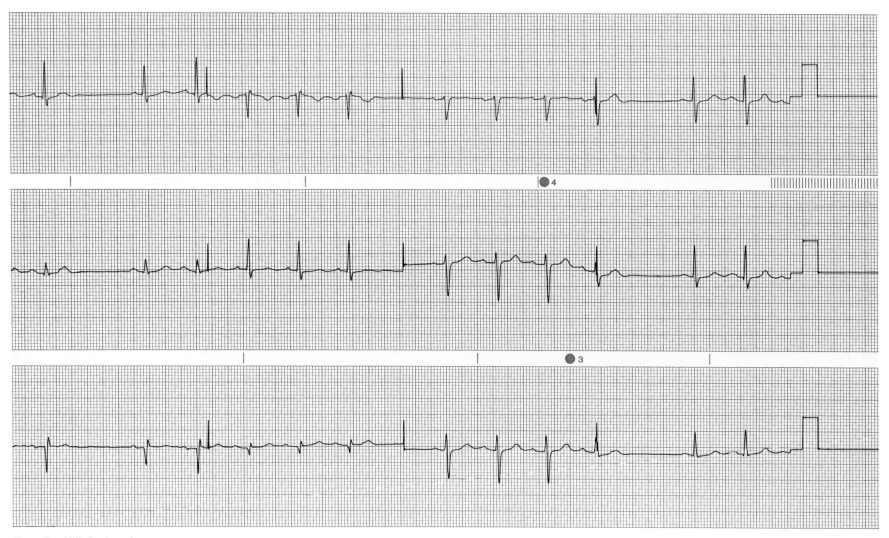

Exercise XIII, Patient 6

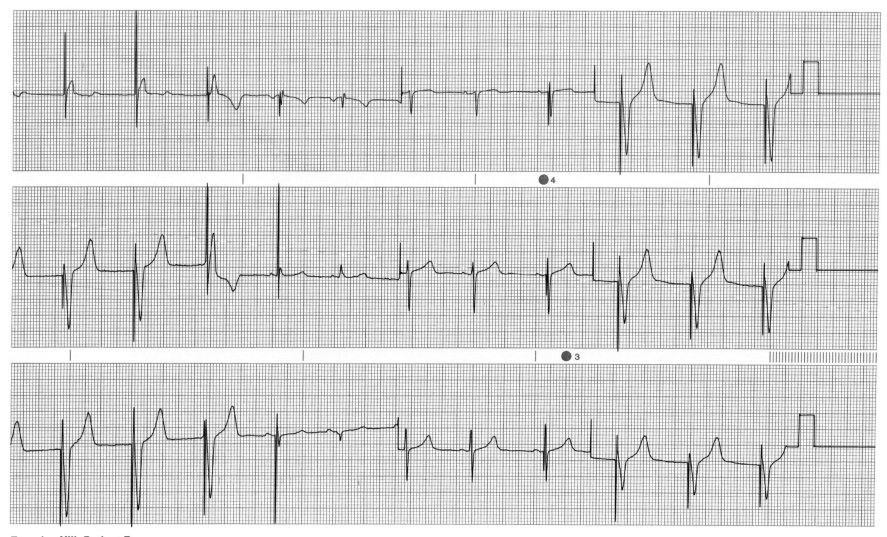

Exercise XIII, Patient 7

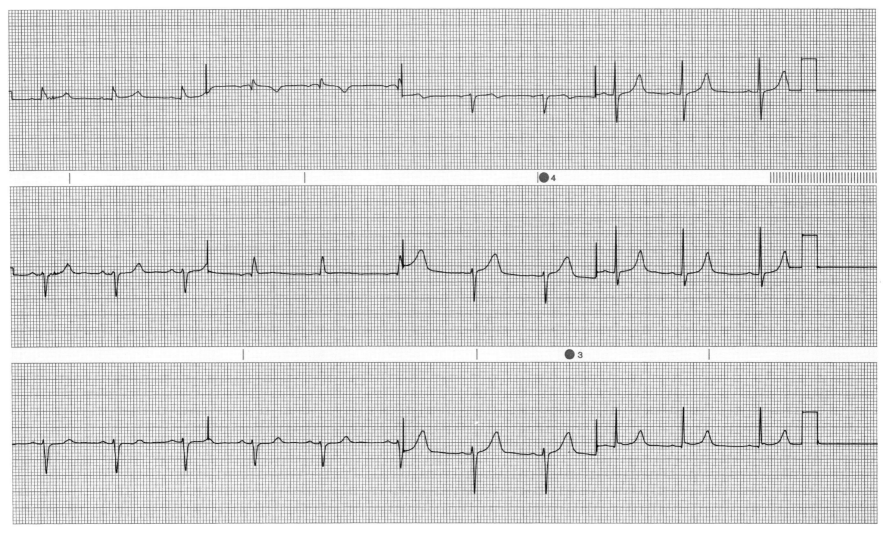

Exercise XIII, Patient 8

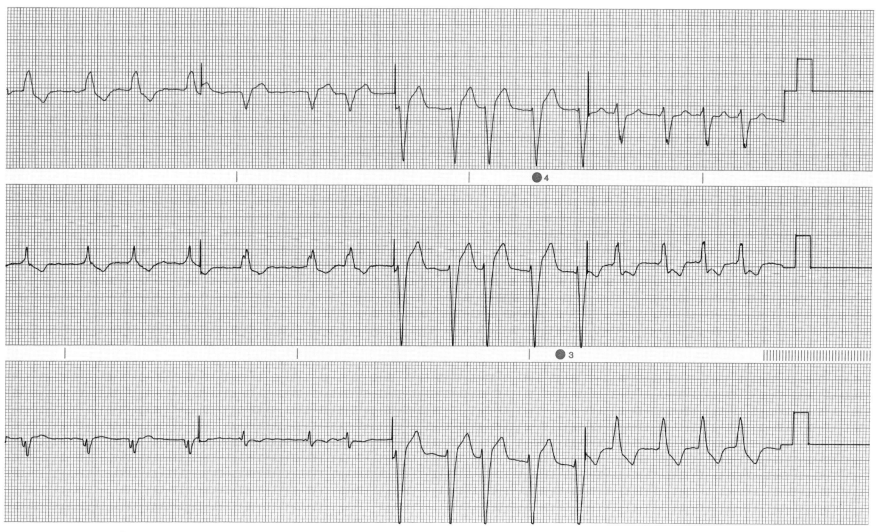

Exercise XIII, Patient 9

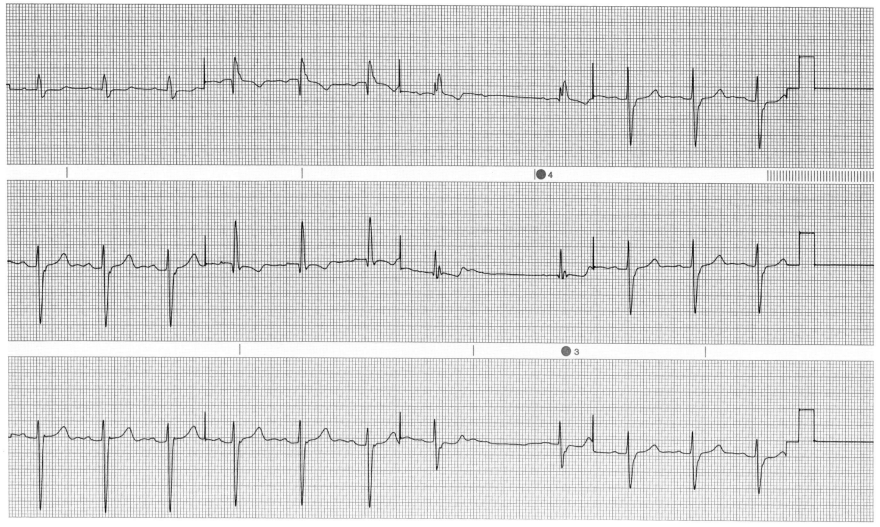

Exercise XIII, Patient 10

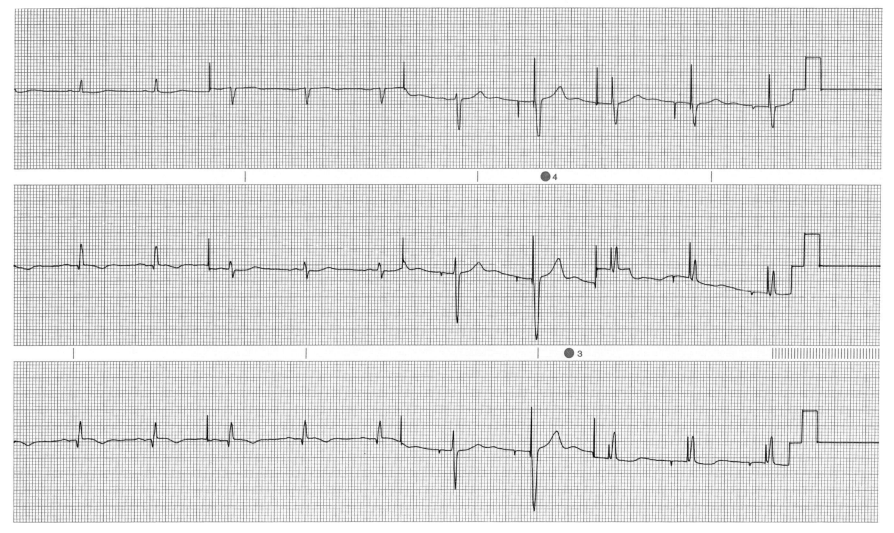

Exercise XIII, Patient 11

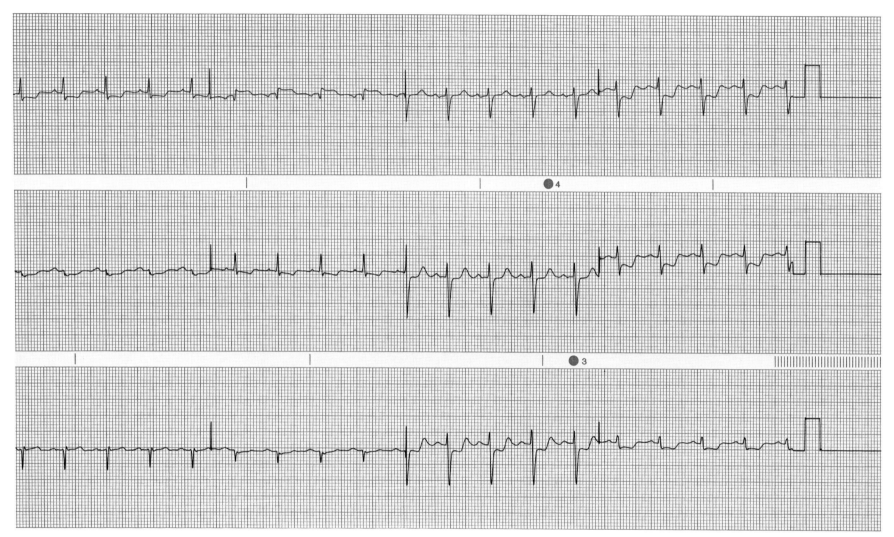

Exercise XIII, Patient 12

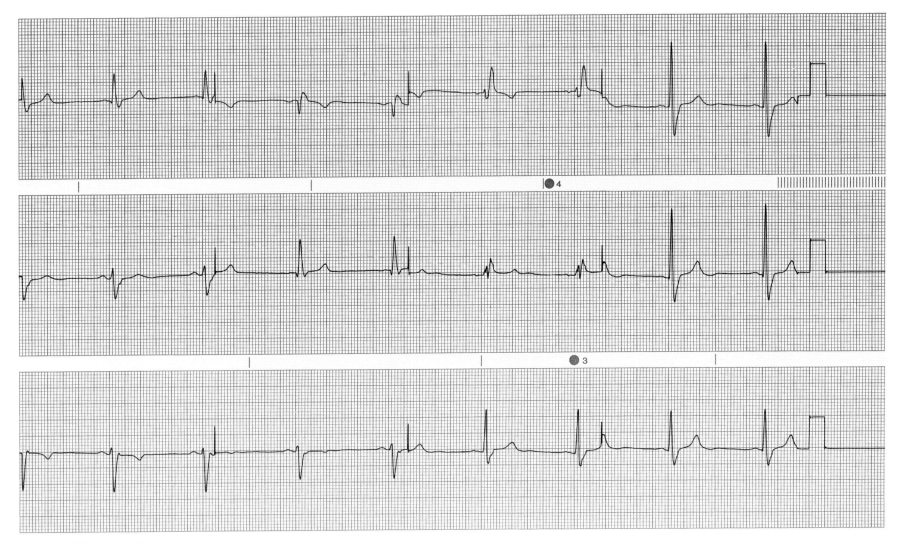

Exercise XIII, Patient 13

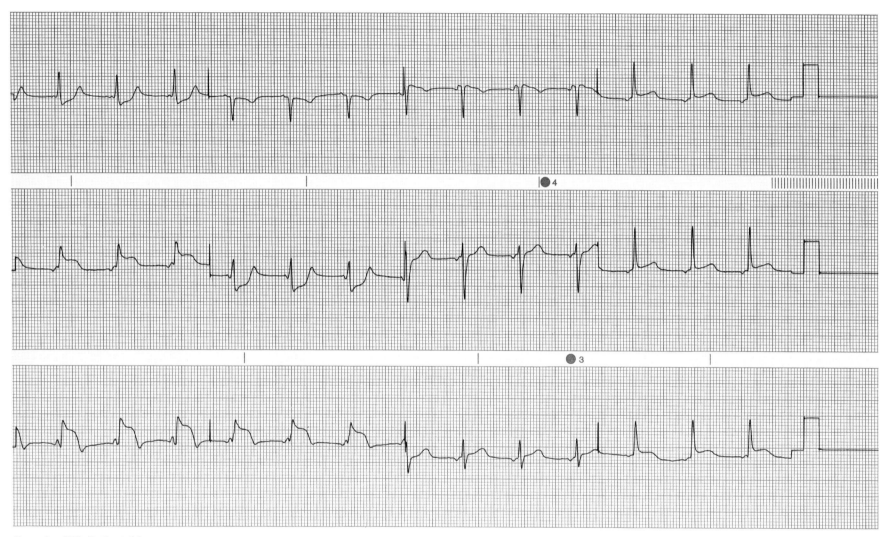

Exercise XIII, Patient 14

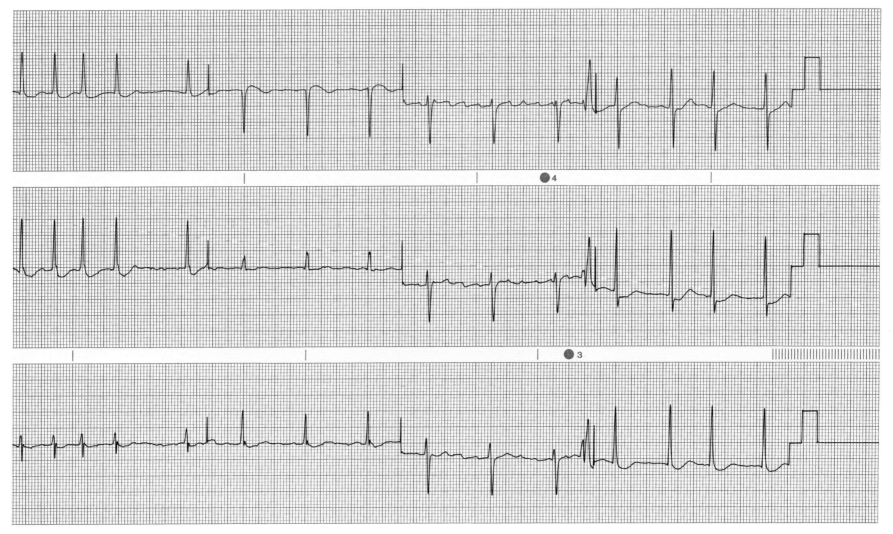

Exercise XIII, Patient 15

1. This electrocardiogram shows a sinus bradycardia with an anterior hemiblock and a right bundle branch block. The right bundle branch block broadens the complex and produces the broad R′ in V_1 and wide terminal S in V_6. Marked left axis deviation with a small Q wave in aV_L establishes the hemiblock. Coded 7, 55, 58, and 86.

2. This shows a sinus rhythm with an old inferoposterior infarction. Q waves are seen in leads II, III, and aV_F with a tall R wave relative to S wave in lead V_1 with an upright T wave. ST segment changes laterally are not specific. Coded 5, 78, 79, 89, and 94.

3. This person has a sinus rhythm with a Wenckebach block. The dropped beats are seen in the second and third panels. There are nonspecific lateral repolarization changes. P waves are wide in lead II, and the terminal portion in V_1 is broadly negative, consistent with left atrial enlargement. There is poor R wave progression, suggesting an anteroseptal infarction. Coded 5, 42, 63, 75, 89, and 94.

4. This electrocardiogram shows a sinus rhythm with a complete left bundle branch block. The complexes are broad, and there are no Q waves in leads I or V_6. Coded 5 and 57.

5. This patient has a sinus rhythm with left axis deviation caused by an anterior hemiblock. Axis is greater than −45 degrees. In lead aV_L there is a small Q wave and an activation delay. There are no other significant changes. Coded 5 and 58.

6. This electrocardiogram shows sinus rhythm with blocked premature atrial contractions (PACs). The block PACs are seen with the first beat of the tracing, since T waves of the first beat are different from the second beat. This distortion is due to a superimposed P wave. The same thing is seen with the last beat in the second panel and the first T wave in the fourth panel. In addition, there are inferior Q waves with broad and relatively prominent negative forces in lead aV_F caused by an old inferior infarction. Coded 5, 10, 78, and 94.

7. This electrocardiogram shows intermittent ventricular pacing. The sinus rhythm and ventricular pacing are nearly isorhythmic with one another. Coded 5, 35, and 37 (and possibly 78, in view of the Q in the aV_F lead). If inferior infarction is diagnosed, then coronary disease (94) also needs to be coded.

8. This shows a sinus rhythm with left axis. In the aV_L lead there are small Q waves and activation abnormalities. The diagnosis is anterior hemiblock. Coded 5 and 58.

9. This is an irregular rhythm. The complex is broad, and there are no Q waves in leads I or V_6. This is atrial fibrillation and a left bundle branch block. Coded 14, 57, and 86.

10. This electrocardiogram shows a sinus rhythm with an intermittent second-degree AV block, right bundle branch block, and an anterior hemiblock. The right bundle branch block is diagnosed by the broad R′ in lead V_1 and the broad terminal S wave in lead V_6. The left axis and Q wave in the aV_L lead are due to anterior hemiblock. Coded 5, 43, 55, 58, and 86.

11. This patient has a sinus rhythm with intermittent AV sequential pacing. There are narrow but relatively deep Q waves associated with 5 mm R waves in the aV_F lead plus T wave changes. This is an inferior myocardial infarction. Coded 7, 35, 38, 78, and 94.

12. This electrocardiogram shows ST segment depression that is horizontal and, in some cases, downsloping. There is a sinus tachycardia; this is most suggestive of subendocardial ischemia. Coded 6, 85, and 94.

13. This is a sinus rhythm with a right bundle branch block and an anterior hemiblock. R′ in V_1 and wide S in V_6 indicate a diagnosis of right bundle branch block. Anterior hemiblock is suggested by left axis deviation and the Q waves in the aV_L lead. Coded 7, 55, and 58.

14. This electrocardiogram shows an ectopic atrial rhythm (diagnosed by the abnormal P axis and short PR interval) and an acute inferior infarction. There is ST segment elevation in leads II, III, aV_F, and V_6 with reciprocal ST changes in leads I and aV_L. Coded 12, 73, 84, and 94.

15. This is coarse atrial fibrillation. There is an aberrant beat, as the last beat in panel 3. This long RR–short RR relationship with aberrancy on the third beat is called Ashman's phenomenon. The ST depression and relatively short QT interval are consistent with digitalis effect. Coded 14, 88, and 61.

Exercise XIV

ANSWER SHEET
Exercise XIV

Patient 1   —— —— —— —— —— —— ——

Patient 2   —— —— —— —— —— —— ——

Patient 3   —— —— —— —— —— —— ——

Patient 4   —— —— —— —— —— —— ——

Patient 5   —— —— —— —— —— —— ——

Patient 6   —— —— —— —— —— —— ——

Patient 7   —— —— —— —— —— —— ——

Patient 8   —— —— —— —— —— —— ——

Patient 9   —— —— —— —— —— —— ——

Patient 10   —— —— —— —— —— —— ——

Patient 11   —— —— —— —— —— —— ——

Patient 12   —— —— —— —— —— —— ——

Patient 13   —— —— —— —— —— —— ——

Patient 14   —— —— —— —— —— —— ——

Patient 15   —— —— —— —— —— —— ——

Electrocardiographic Diagnostic Coding Sheet

General Features
1. Normal ECG
2. Normal ECG, variant
3. Misplaced leads
4. Electrical alternans

Sinus Rhythms
5. Normal sinus
6. Sinus tachycardia
7. Sinus bradycardia
8. Sinus arrhythmia
9. Sinus pause or arrest

Atrial Rhythms
10. Premature atrial contractions (PAC)
11. Aberrant PAC
12. Ectopic atrial rhythm
13. Atrial tachycardia with AV block
14. Atrial fibrillation
15. Atrial flutter
16. Multifocal atrial tachycardia
17. Dual atrial rhythms

AV Junctional Rhythms
18. Premature junctional beats (PJB)
19. Aberrant PJB
20. Junctional beat or rhythm
21. AV junctional rhythm with retrograde atrial activation
22. Supraventricular tachycardia

Ventricular Rhythms
23. Premature ventricular contractions (PVC), unifocal
24. PVC, multifocal
25. PVC, couplets/triplets
26. PVC, R-on-T

27. Ventricular tachycardia
28. Idioventricular rhythm
29. Ventricular fibrillation
30. Ventricular escape beat or rhythm
31. Ventricular fusion beat or rhythm
32. Ventricular capture beat during VT
33. Torsades de pointes

Pacemaker Rhythms
34. Fixed rate
35. Demand
36. Atrial pacing
37. Ventricular pacing
38. Dual chamber pacing
39. Failure to sense
40. Failure to capture

AV Conduction Abnormalities
41. 1° AV block
42. Wenckebach (Mobitz I) AV block
43. 2° AV block (Mobitz II)
44. Fixed 2° AV block, 2:1, 4:1, etc.
45. Complete heart block
46. Variable AV block
47. Preexcitation (WPW)

AV - VA Interactions
48. Fusion beat
49. Echo beat
50. AV dissociation
51. Isorhythmic AV dissociation

Intraventricular Conduction Abnormalities
52. Left axis

53. Right axis
54. Incomplete RBBB
55. Complete RBBB
56. Incomplete LBBB
57. Complete LBBB
58. Anterior hemiblock
59. Posterior hemiblock
60. Nonspecific IVCD
61. Arrhythmia related aberrancy
62. Intermittent IVCD/BBB

Chamber Enlargement
63. Left atrial enlargement
64. Right atrial enlargement
65. Bi-atrial enlargement
66. LVH - voltage
67. LVH - voltage plus repolarization changes
68. RVH
69. Biventricular hypertrophy

Myocardial Infarction

Recent/Acute
70. Anteroseptal
71. Anterior
72. Lateral
73. Inferior
74. Posterior

Old/Uncertain Age
75. Anteroseptal
76. Anterior
77. Lateral
78. Inferior
79. Posterior

Repolarization Changes
80. Possible LV aneurysm
81. Non-Q wave infarction

82. Early repolarization
83. Persistent juvenile T wave
84. ST-T wave changes of acute injury
85. ST-T wave changes of acute ischemia
86. ST-T wave changes of hypertrophy or altered intraventricular conduction (secondary repolarization changes)
87. ST-T wave changes of pericarditis
88. ST changes due to digitalis effect
89. Nonspecific ST-T wave changes
90. Postectopic T wave changes
91. Peaked T waves
92. Prolonged QT interval
93. Prominent U waves

Clinical Problems
94. Coronary artery disease
95. Congenital heart disease
96. Mitral valve disease
97. Hyperkalemia
98. Hypokalemia
99. Hypercalcemia
100. Hypocalcemia
101. Digitalis toxicity
102. CNS event
103. Motion artifact
104. Dextrocardia
105. Cardiac tamponade
106. Cardiac transplant
107. Chronic lung disease

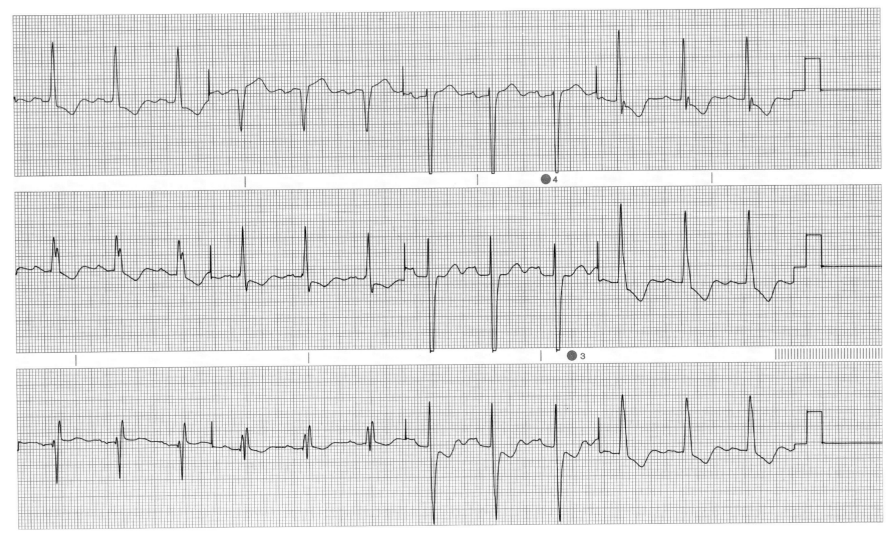

Exercise XIV, Patient 1

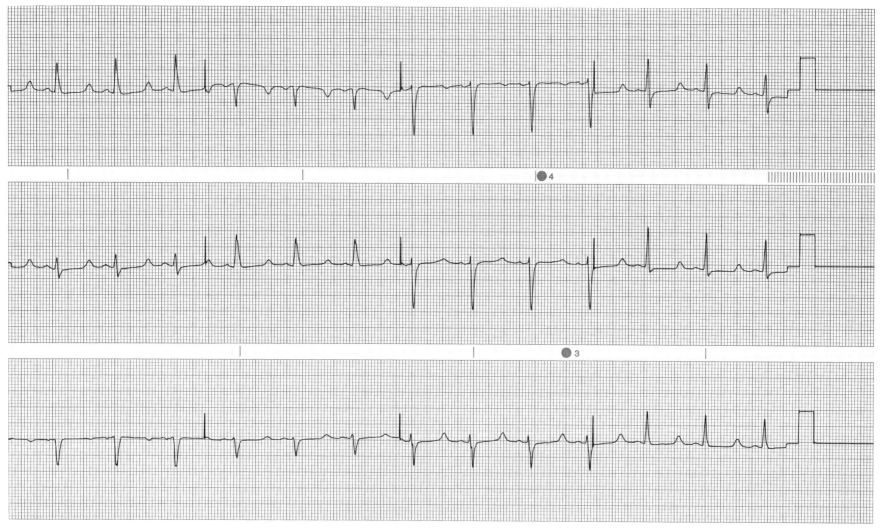

Exercise XIV, Patient 2

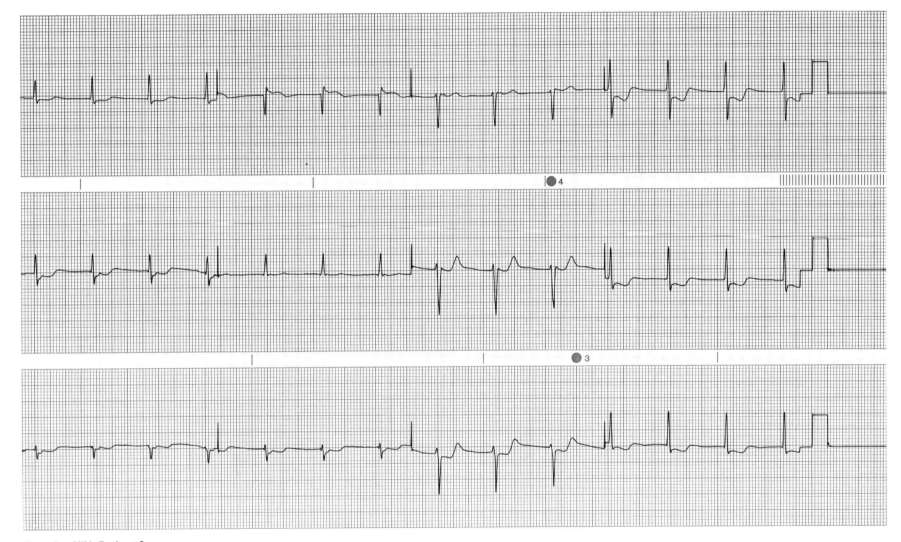

Exercise XIV, Patient 3

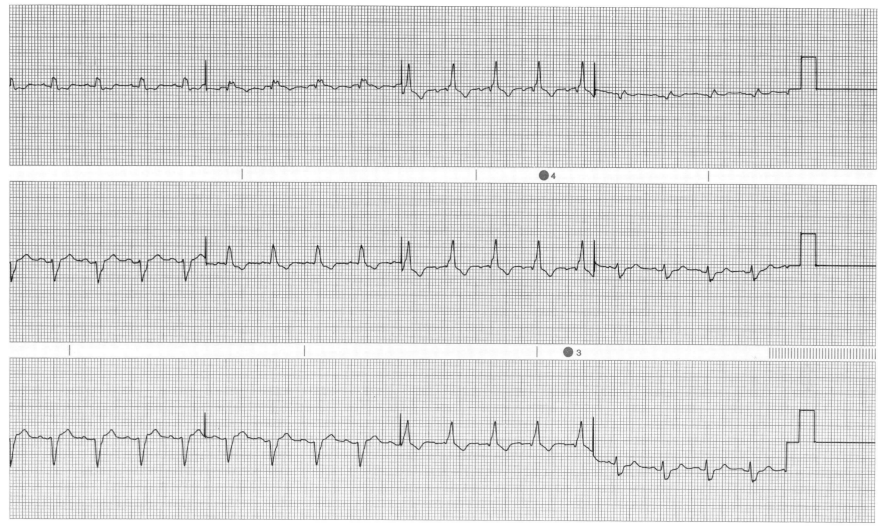

Exercise XIV, Patient 4

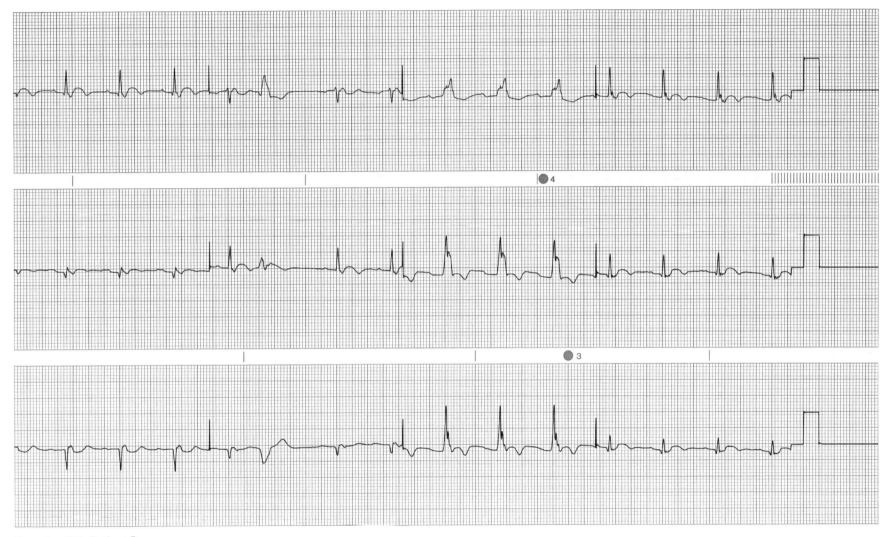

Exercise XIV, Patient 5

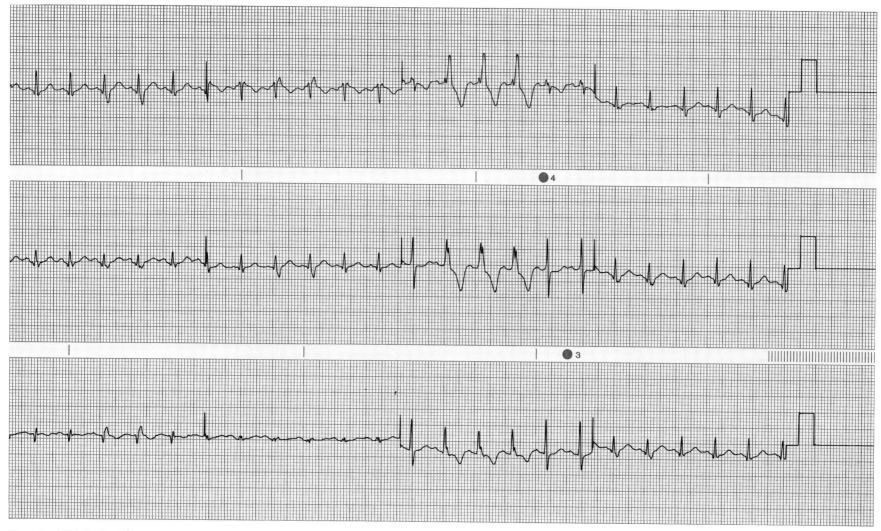

Exercise XIV, Patient 6

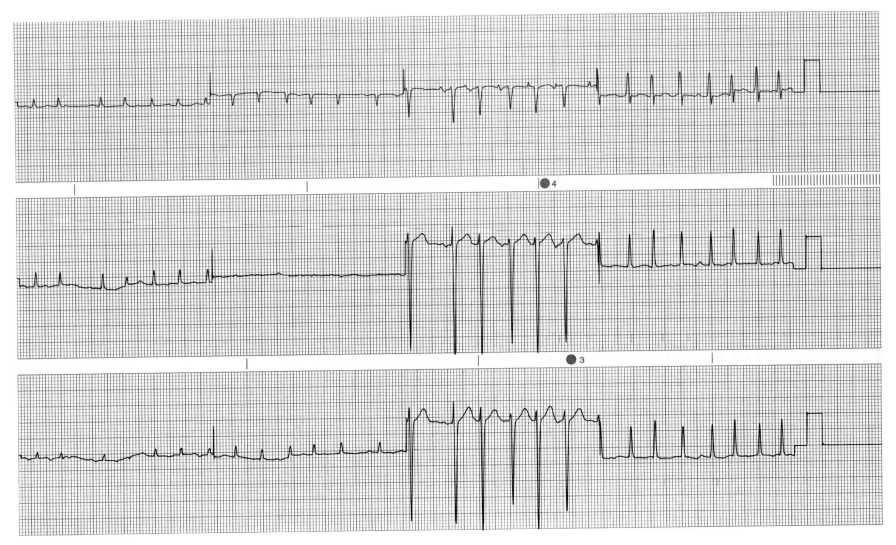

Exercise XIV, Patient 7

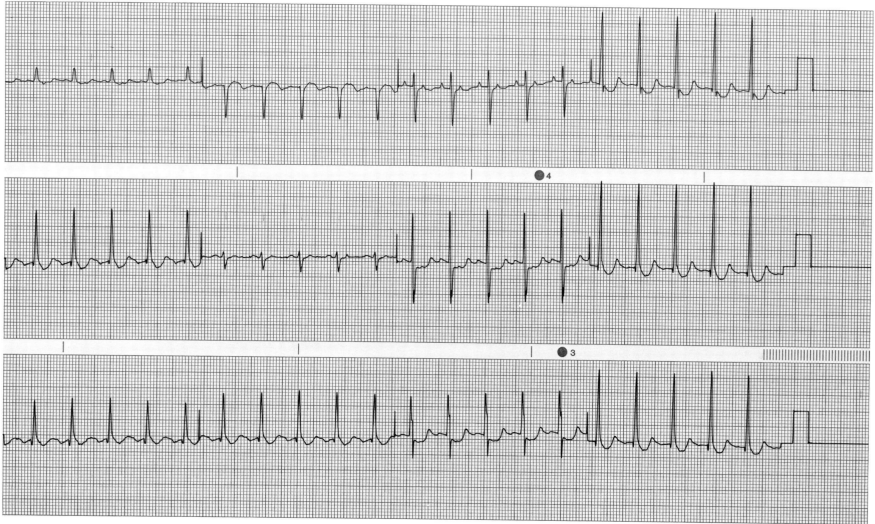

Exercise XIV, Patient 8

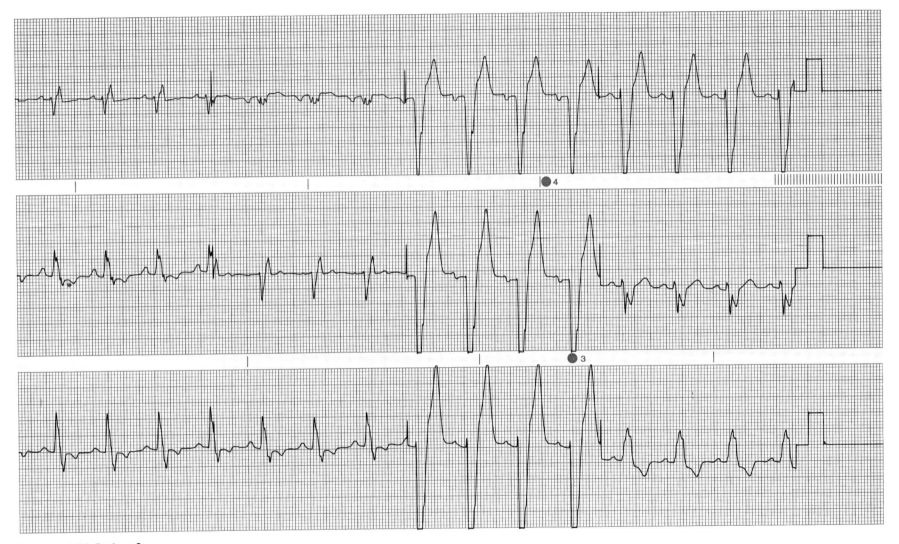

Exercise XIV, Patient 9

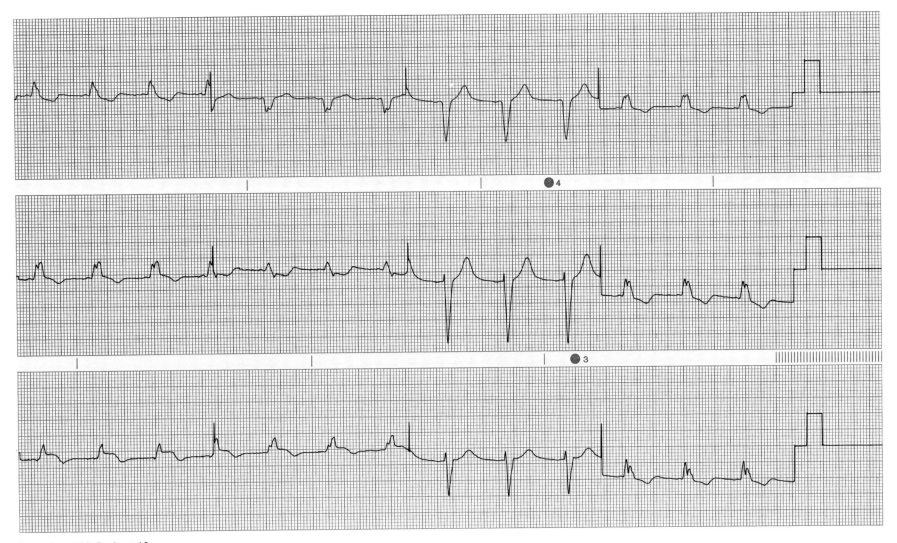

Exercise XIV, Patient 10

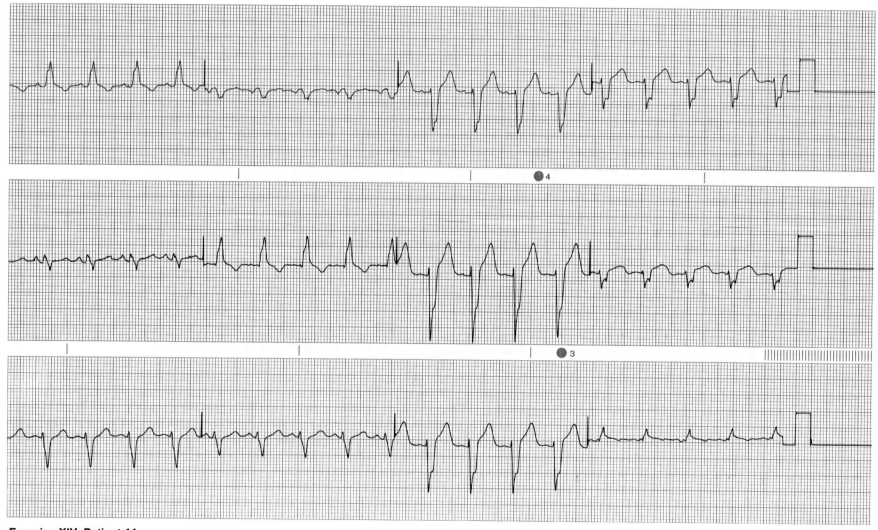

Exercise XIV, Patient 11

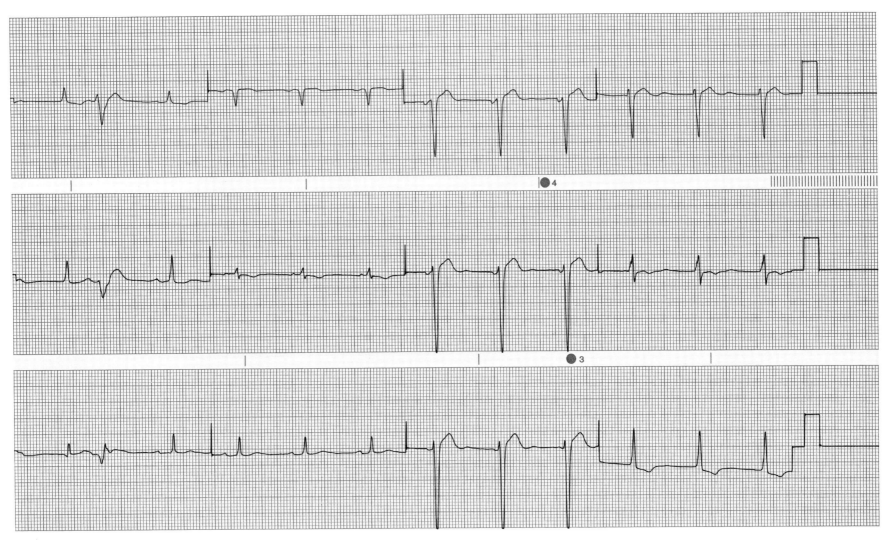

Exercise XIV, Patient 12

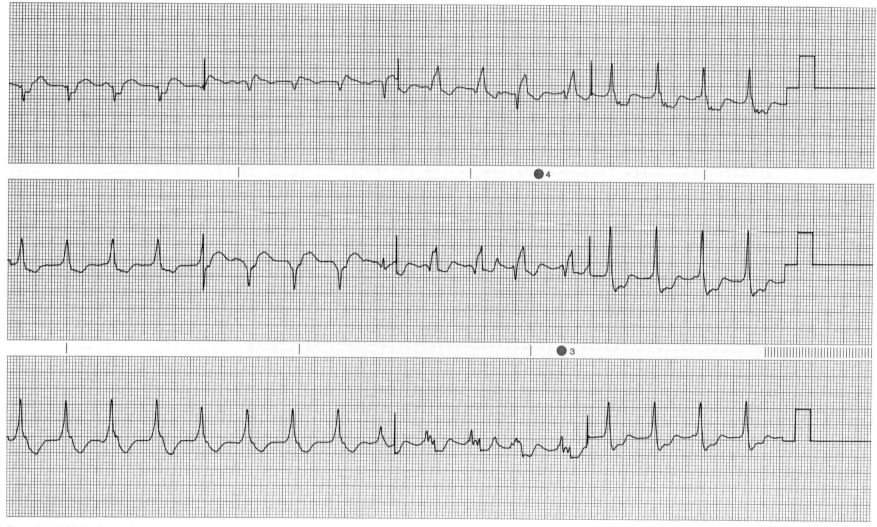

Exercise XIV, Patient 13

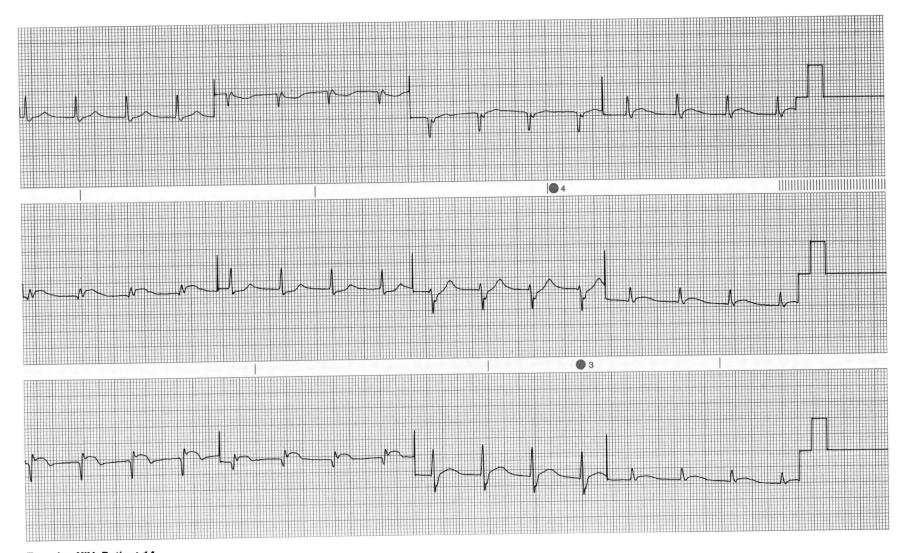

Exercise XIV, Patient 14

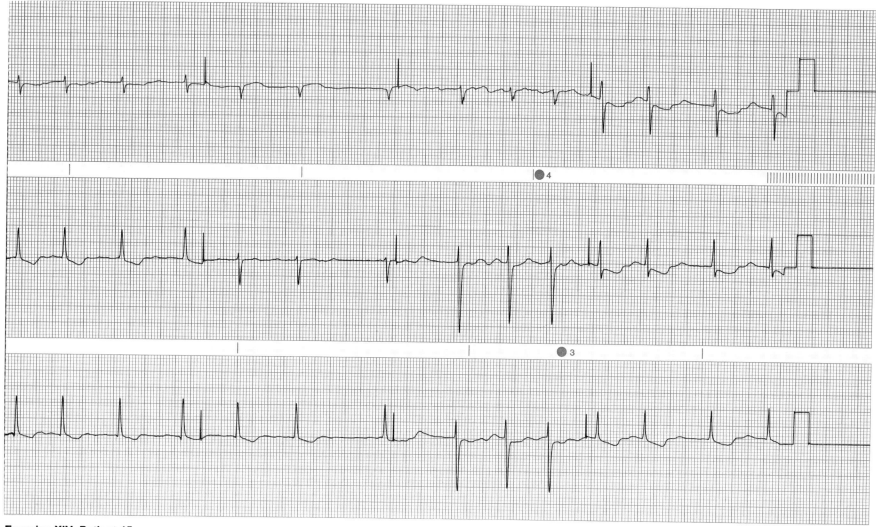

Exercise XIV, Patient 15

1. This electrocardiogram is a left bundle branch block, possibly from ventricular hypertrophy. (The QRS complex is >120 milliseconds. There are no septal Q waves in leads I or V_6.) In addition, there is left atrial enlargement with broad notched P waves in leads I and II, and broad, terminally negative P waves in lead V_1. The PR interval is prolonged. Coded 5, 41, 57, 63, and 86.

2. This electrocardiogram shows a sinus rhythm with a very long QT interval but a normal-appearing T wave, indicating hypocalcemia. Coded 5, 92, and 100.

3. This has a nodal rhythm with retrograde activation of the atria. There are also ST segment depression and nonspecific T wave changes. Coded 21 and 89.

4. This patient has a complete right bundle branch block with marked left axis, consistent with anterior hemiblock and Q waves in leads V_1 to V_4 caused by anteroseptal infarction. Coded 5, 55, 58, 75, and 94.

5. This electrocardiogram shows a sinus rhythm, right bundle branch block, and an inferior infarction. Inferior infarction is diagnosed by the Q waves in aV_F. This is supported by Q waves in leads II and III. The right bundle branch block is diagnosed by the width of the complex, the broad terminal S in V_6, and the prominent R′ in lead V_1. There is also a premature ventricular contraction (PVC) seen in the second panel. Coded 5, 23, 55, 78, and 94.

6. This electrocardiogram shows sinus rhythm with intermittent right bundle branch block. This conduction defect is seen in the third panel and in the third and fourth beats of the first panel. Coded 6 and 62 (and possibly 55).

7. This patient has multifocal atrial tachycardia, established by three atrial foci. Changes of ventricular hypertrophy, right or left, are not seen. The ST-T wave changes are not specific. Coded 16 and 89.

8. This electrocardiogram shows atrial tachycardia with a 2:1 AV block. There is ST segment depression, scooping in quality, with a relatively short QT interval, suggesting digitalis effect. Coded 13 and 88 (and possibly 101).

9. This patient has a sinus rhythm, left atrial enlargement, right axis, and a left bundle branch block. There are no Q waves in leads I or V_6, and the QRS complex is >0.12 second. The P wave in lead V_1 is broadly negative in its terminal portions. Coded 5, 53, 57, 63, and 86.

10. This electrocardiogram shows a left bundle branch block, indicated by the prolonged QRS complex and no septal Q waves in leads I or V_6. This is an instance in which the possibility of an acute injury can be raised in view of the ST segment elevation and T wave changes in the inferior leads. This is a less specific call, however. Coded 5 and 57 (and possibly 84).

11. This electrocardiogram also shows a left bundle branch block from which an additional diagnosis can be made. The QRS complex is broad, and there are no Q waves in leads I or V_6. There is generalized ST segment elevation consistent with pericarditis. This also is a less specific call but seems reasonable in view of the diffuse nature of the ST segment elevation. Coded 6, 57, and 87.

12. This patient has sinus and junctional rhythms that show isorhythmic dissociation. In addition, there is a premature ventricular beat as well as nonspecific lateral changes. Coded 5, 20, 23, 51, and 89.

13. This electrocardiogram shows a wide complex tachycardia. It looks like a right bundle branch block but, in fact, is ventricular tachycardia. There is AV dissociation as well as a fusion beat seen in the third panel. Coded 5, 27, 31, and 50.

14. This patient has an acute inferior infarction with a junctional rhythm. There is ST segment elevation and early T wave inversion in leads II, III, and aV_F. Coded 20, 73, 84, and 94.

15. This shows atrial fibrillation, right axis deviation, ST segment depression with prominent U waves, and T-U fusion consistent with hypokalemia. Coded 14, 53, 93, and 98.

Exercise XV

ANSWER SHEET
Exercise XV

Patient 1 —— —— —— —— —— —— —— ——

Patient 2 —— —— —— —— —— —— —— ——

Patient 3 —— —— —— —— —— —— —— ——

Patient 4 —— —— —— —— —— —— —— ——

Patient 5 —— —— —— —— —— —— —— ——

Patient 6 —— —— —— —— —— —— —— ——

Patient 7 —— —— —— —— —— —— —— ——

Patient 8 —— —— —— —— —— —— —— ——

Patient 9 —— —— —— —— —— —— —— ——

Patient 10 —— —— —— —— —— —— —— ——

Patient 11 —— —— —— —— —— —— —— ——

Patient 12 —— —— —— —— —— —— —— ——

Patient 13 —— —— —— —— —— —— —— ——

Patient 14 —— —— —— —— —— —— —— ——

Patient 15 —— —— —— —— —— —— —— ——

Electrocardiographic Diagnostic Coding Sheet

General Features
1. Normal ECG
2. Normal ECG, variant
3. Misplaced leads
4. Electrical alternans

Sinus Rhythms
5. Normal sinus
6. Sinus tachycardia
7. Sinus bradycardia
8. Sinus arrhythmia
9. Sinus pause or arrest

Atrial Rhythms
10. Premature atrial contractions (PAC)
11. Aberrant PAC
12. Ectopic atrial rhythm
13. Atrial tachycardia with AV block
14. Atrial fibrillation
15. Atrial flutter
16. Multifocal atrial tachycardia
17. Dual atrial rhythms

AV Junctional Rhythms
18. Premature junctional beats (PJB)
19. Aberrant PJB
20. Junctional beat or rhythm
21. AV junctional rhythm with retrograde atrial activation
22. Supraventricular tachycardia

Ventricular Rhythms
23. Premature ventricular contractions (PVC), unifocal
24. PVC, multifocal
25. PVC, couplets/triplets
26. PVC, R-on-T

27. Ventricular tachycardia
28. Idioventricular rhythm
29. Ventricular fibrillation
30. Ventricular escape beat or rhythm
31. Ventricular fusion beat or rhythm
32. Ventricular capture beat during VT
33. Torsades de pointes

Pacemaker Rhythms
34. Fixed rate
35. Demand
36. Atrial pacing
37. Ventricular pacing
38. Dual chamber pacing
39. Failure to sense
40. Failure to capture

AV Conduction Abnormalities
41. 1° AV block
42. Wenckebach (Mobitz I) AV block
43. 2° AV block (Mobitz II)
44. Fixed 2° AV block, 2:1, 4:1, etc.
45. Complete heart block
46. Variable AV block
47. Preexcitation (WPW)

AV - VA Interactions
48. Fusion beat
49. Echo beat
50. AV dissociation
51. Isorhythmic AV dissociation

Intraventricular Conduction Abnormalities
52. Left axis

53. Right axis
54. Incomplete RBBB
55. Complete RBBB
56. Incomplete LBBB
57. Complete LBBB
58. Anterior hemiblock
59. Posterior hemiblock
60. Nonspecific IVCD
61. Arrhythmia related aberrancy
62. Intermittent IVCD/BBB

Chamber Enlargement
63. Left atrial enlargement
64. Right atrial enlargement
65. Bi-atrial enlargement
66. LVH - voltage
67. LVH - voltage plus repolarization changes
68. RVH
69. Biventricular hypertrophy

Myocardial Infarction

Recent/Acute
70. Anteroseptal
71. Anterior
72. Lateral
73. Inferior
74. Posterior

Old/Uncertain Age
75. Anteroseptal
76. Anterior
77. Lateral
78. Inferior
79. Posterior

Repolarization Changes
80. Possible LV aneurysm
81. Non-Q wave infarction

82. Early repolarization
83. Persistent juvenile T wave
84. ST-T wave changes of acute injury
85. ST-T wave changes of acute ischemia
86. ST-T wave changes of hypertrophy or altered intraventricular conduction (secondary repolarization changes)
87. ST-T wave changes of pericarditis
88. ST changes due to digitalis effect
89. Nonspecific ST-T wave changes
90. Postectopic T wave changes
91. Peaked T waves
92. Prolonged QT interval
93. Prominent U waves

Clinical Problems
94. Coronary artery disease
95. Congenital heart disease
96. Mitral valve disease
97. Hyperkalemia
98. Hypokalemia
99. Hypercalcemia
100. Hypocalcemia
101. Digitalis toxicity
102. CNS event
103. Motion artifact
104. Dextrocardia
105. Cardiac tamponade
106. Cardiac transplant
107. Chronic lung disease

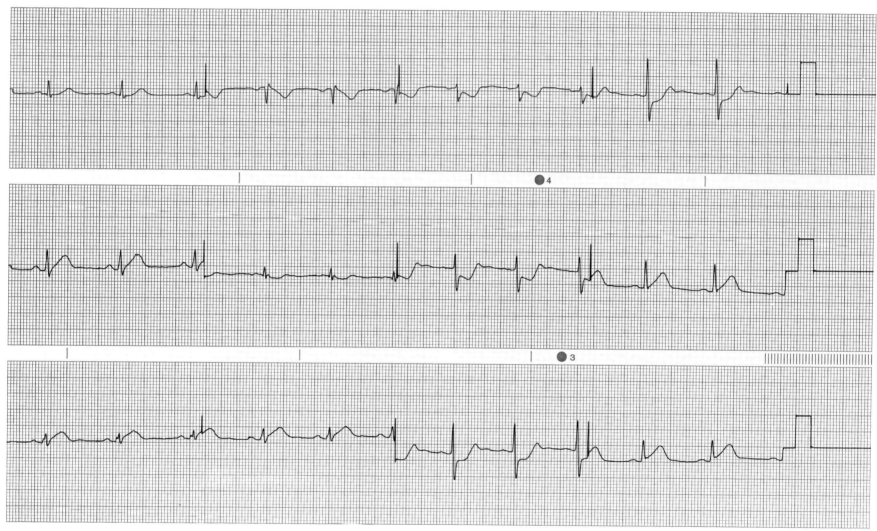

Exercise XV, Patient 1

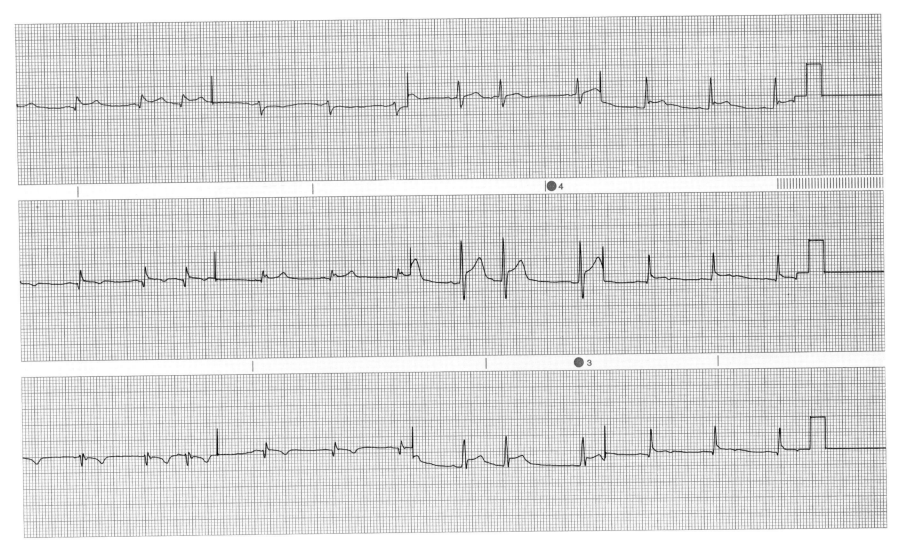

Exercise XV, Patient 2

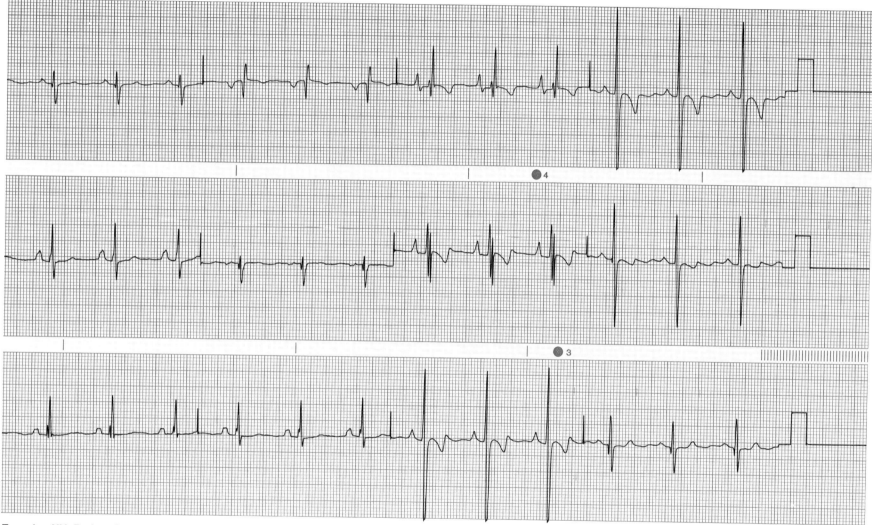

Exercise XV, Patient 3

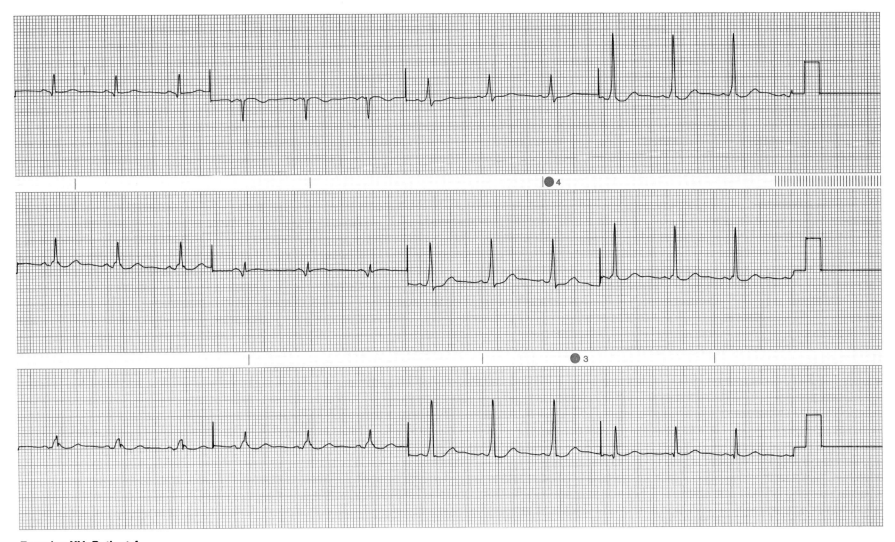

Exercise XV, Patient 4

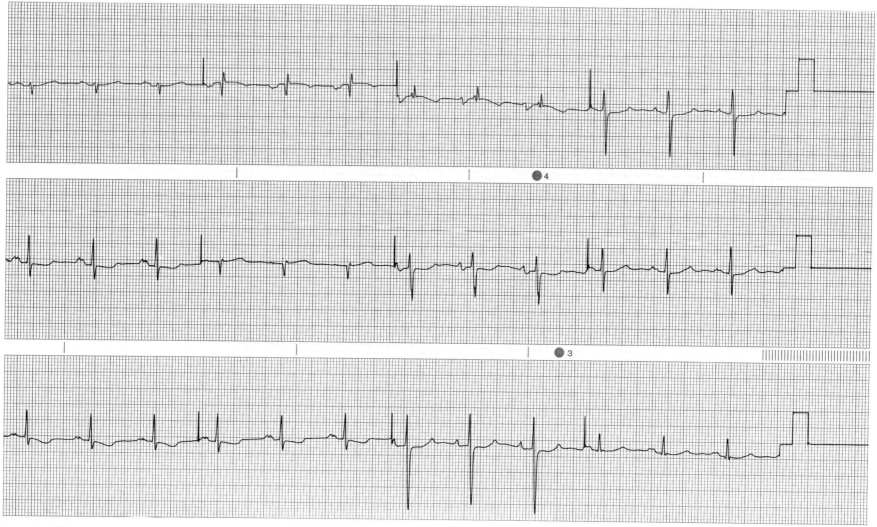

Exercise XV, Patient 5

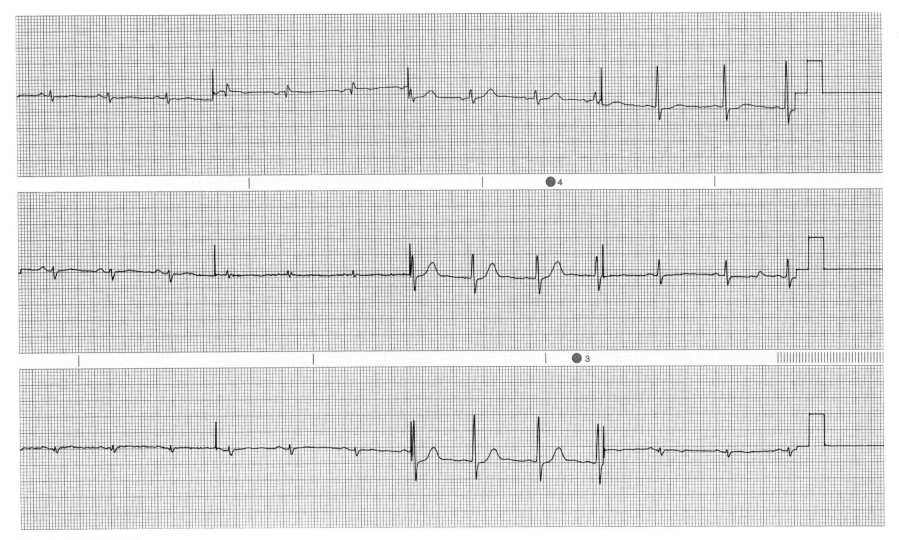

Exercise XV, Patient 6

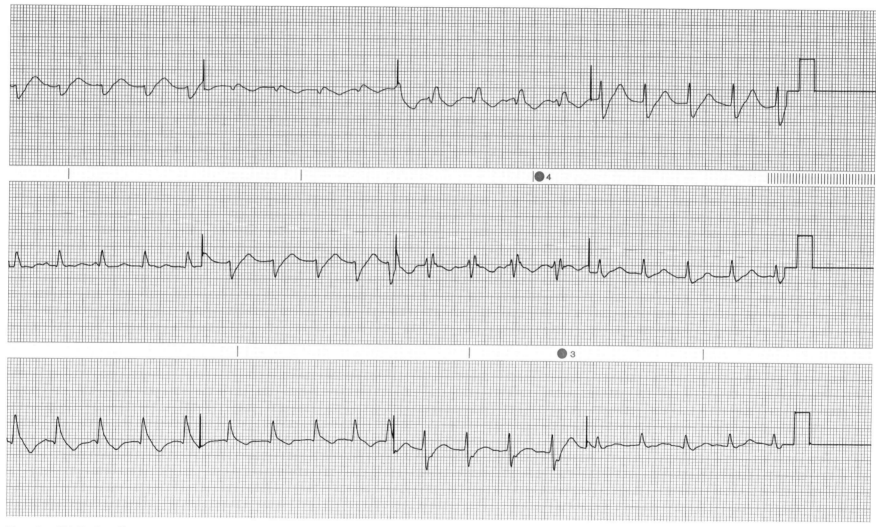

Exercise XV, Patient 7

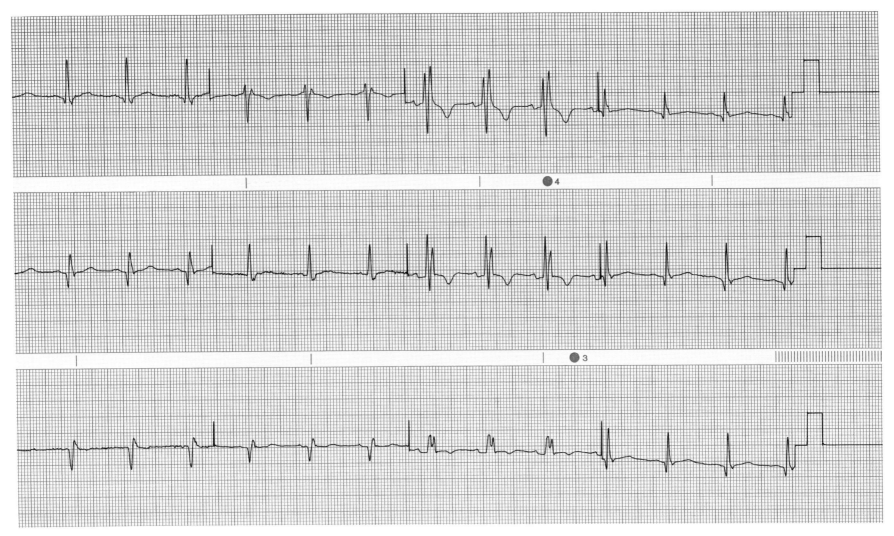

Exercise XV, Patient 8

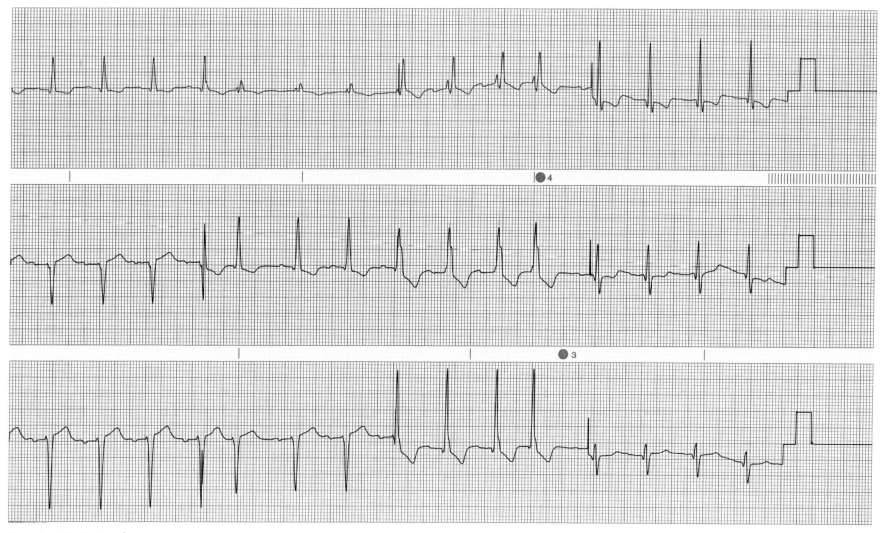

Exercise XV, Patient 9

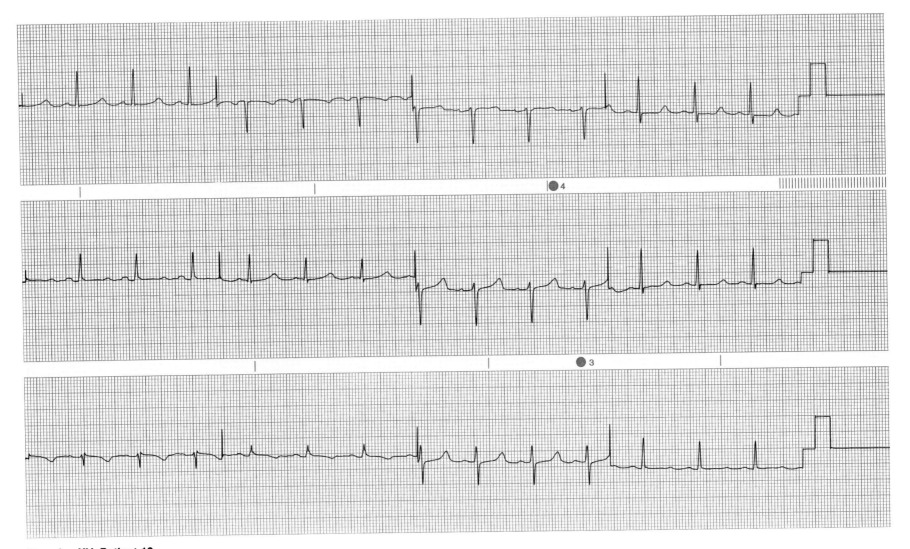

Exercise XV, Patient 10

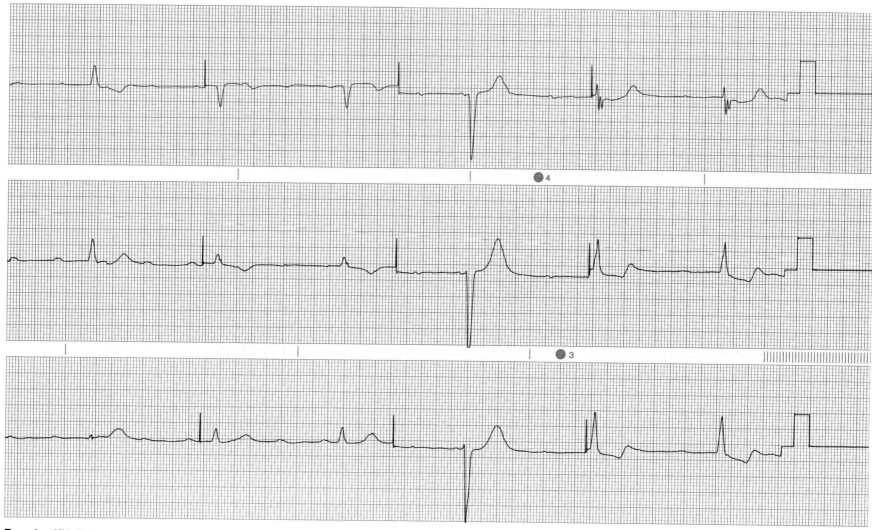

Exercise XV, Patient 11

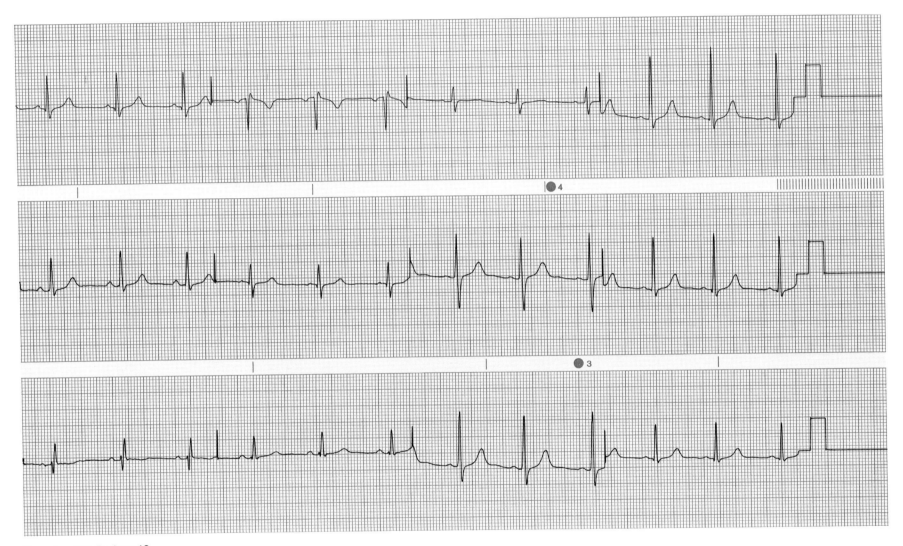

Exercise XV, Patient 12

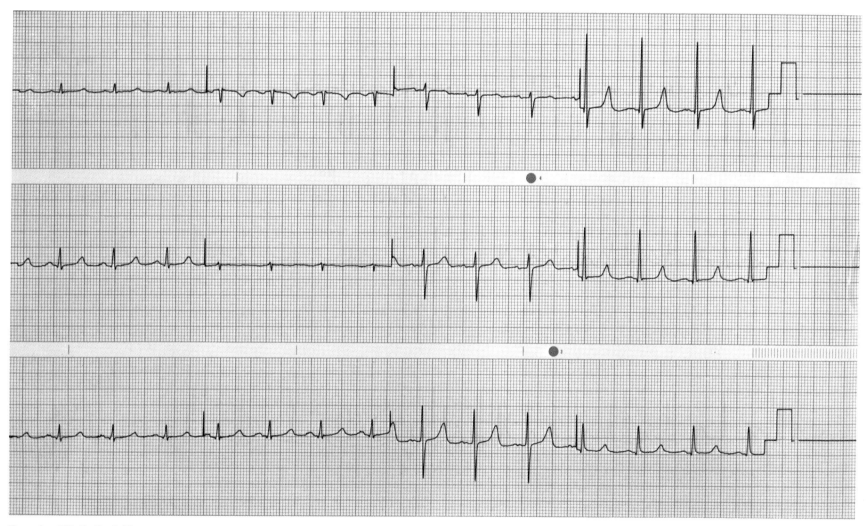

Exercise XV, Patient 13

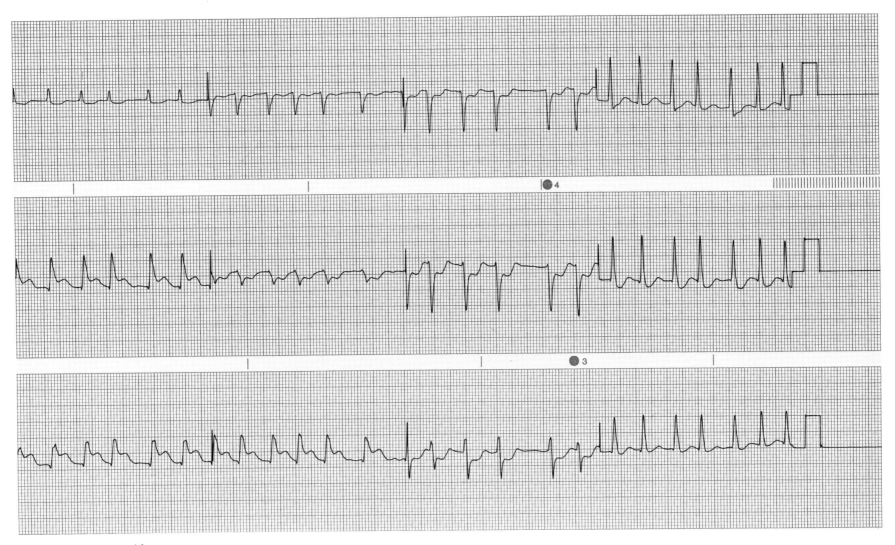

Exercise XV, Patient 14

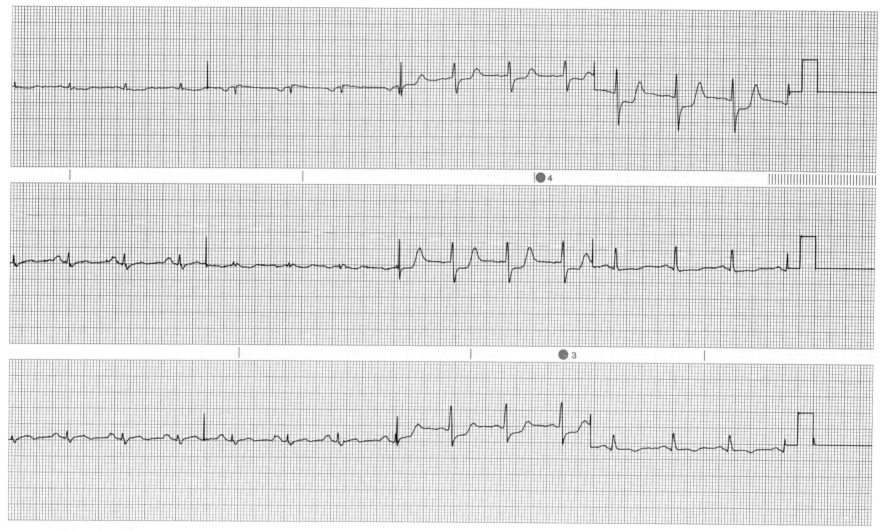

Exercise XV, Patient 15

1. This is an acute inferior infarction. There is minimal ST segment elevation in the inferior leads, but the T waves have a hyperacute quality, being symmetric and broad-based, and there are reciprocal changes in leads V_1 to V_4. Coded 5, 73, 84, and 94.

2. This electrocardiogram shows a posterolateral infarction with pericarditis. Premature atrial contractions (PACs) are seen in the first and third panels. Coded 5, 10, 79, 87, and 94.

3. This shows right ventricular hypertrophy and right atrial enlargement. The axis is to the right, an rsR' in lead V_1 with $R' > S$ and T wave inversion. The P waves in leads V_1 and II are narrow but prominent. The $R:S$ ratio in lead V_5 is also consistent with right ventricular hypertrophy. Coded 5, 54, 64, and 68.

4. This tracing has a prominent R wave in lead V_1, which might represent a posterior infarction or right ventricular hypertrophy. In fact, it is Wolff-Parkinson-White syndrome. Coded 5 and 47.

5. This electrocardiogram has a sinus rhythm. There is left atrial enlargement with notched P waves in lead II and a broadly negative terminal P wave in lead V_1. An rsR' pattern with $R' > S$ and T wave inversion in lead V_1 raise the possibility of right ventricular hypertrophy. This is right ventricular hypertrophy and left atrial enlargement probably caused by chronic mitral valvular disease. Coded 5, 53, 54, 63, 68, 86, and 96.

6. This is a posterolateral infarction. The R wave is greater than S wave in lead V_1, and the T wave is upright. There is a qrS in lead V_6, which by itself would not be diagnostic but in light of the posterior infarct in lead V_1 suggests posterolateral involvement. Coded 5, 77, 79, and 94.

7. This shows sinus tachycardia with an accelerated nodal rhythm dissociated from the sinus mechanism. There is a right bundle branch block with broad R' in lead V_1 and terminal S wave in lead V_6. There is ST segment elevation in leads III and aV_F with T wave inversion, suggesting acute inferior infarction. In addition, the QRS complex is generally broadened with a smooth merging of the terminal portion of the S wave and the T wave, especially evident in leads V_4 and V_5, which raises the possibility of hyperkalemia. Coded 6, 20, 51, 55, 73, 84, and 94 (and possibly 97).

8. This is a sinus rhythm with a right bundle branch block and inferior and lateral infarcts. Q waves in leads V_4 to V_6 are wide and significant. Inferior Q waves are broad and deep. Coded 5, 55, 77, 78, and 94.

9. This electrocardiogram shows a sinus rhythm with a right bundle branch block, anterior hemiblock, and lateral infarction from coronary artery disease. The right bundle and anterior hemiblock are fairly obvious with the broad R' wave and deep terminal S wave in lead V_6, the axis markedly to the left, and a small Q wave with some secondary activation abnormalities in the aV_L lead. In addition, the Q waves in leads V_4 to V_6 are significant. Occasional PACs are present. Coded 5, 10, 55, 58, 77, and 94.

10. This electrocardiogram shows a sinus rhythm with a long QT interval and a normal T wave, indicating hypocalcemia. Coded 5, 92, and 100.

11. This electrocardiogram shows a sinus rhythm with complete heart block and a ventricular escape rhythm. Coded 5, 30, and 45.

12. This is a normal electrocardiogram with marked counterclockwise rotation. From an electrocardiographic point of view, this might be a posterior infarct. Clinically, it was a young patient with no risk factors for coronary heart disease. Coded 1 and 5.

13. This electrocardiogram shows a sinus rhythm. There is symmetric prominence of the T waves, especially in the lateral precordial leads, as well as relative prolongation of the QT interval. This raises the possibility of hypocalcemia and hyperkalemia, which was the case in this chronic dialysis patient. Coded 5, 91, 92, 97, and 100.

14. This electrocardiogram shows atrial fibrillation (an irregularly irregular ventricular response) and an acute inferior infarct with ST segment elevation in leads II, III, and aV_F and reciprocal depressions in leads aV_L and V_1 to V_3. Coded 14, 73, 84, and 94.

15. This shows prominent R waves in leads V_1 and V_2. There is ST segment depression that is horizontal in leads V_2 and V_4. This could be an acute posterior infarction or an old posterior infarction with subendocardial ischemia. Coded either 5, 74, 84, and 94 or 5, 79, 85, and 94.

Index

Note: Pages in *italics* indicate illustrations.